Healing the Eye the Natural Way

Alternative Medicine
and
Macular Degeneration

Healing the Eye the Natural Way

Alternative Medicine
and
Macular Degeneration

Edward Kondrot MD

Nutritional Research Press
1-877-341-2703

The information in this book is meant to complement standard medical care. Any unusual, sudden, or severe symptoms should be evaluated by an ophthalmologist. The recommendations made in this book, while generally safe and non-toxic, may affect people differently. Therefore it is recommended that individuals with serious eye disease be under the care of a physician.

Cover Design by: Behar Fengal Design

This book is dedicated to my sons
Philip, Ryan, and Sean
May they have clear vision all their lives.

Acknowledgments

Why another book dealing with alternative medicine and vision problems? I felt there was a need for a book that goes beyond nutrition, vitamin and mineral therapy for the treatment of macular degeneration. Over 20 years of practice have convinced me that there are alternative therapies that can be of great value in the treatment of this disabling condition. I want to share with the reader important information regarding vision therapy, homeopathy, Chelation and Microcurrent Stimulation that can change the life and sight of many people.

I thank my parents who have always encouraged me to question and to explore new ideas.

I also want to thank the many ophthalmologists who have helped me in my traditional training: Chandra Reshmi, Harold Scheie, Richard Stout and Laura Pallan.

I would also like to thank those ophthalmologists who are also incorporating alternative medicine in their practices: Dahlia Hirsch, Harold Byer, George Khouri and Debra Banker.

I am a grateful to all of my homeopathic teachers: Bill Gray, Karl Robinson, Roger Morrison, Nancy Herrick, Jonathan Shore, Ananda Zaran, Jayesh Shah, Rajan Sankaran and A. U. Ramakrishnan. Todd Rowe, Bill Mann, and Frannie Berez, my homeopathic friends, have helped me in many ways over the years. My gratitude to them.

I am grateful to my business coach, Vance Caesar, who helped transform my ideas into this book.

I would also like to thank those people involved with Microcurrent stimulation in particular Joel Rosen and Damon Miller.

Those who deepened my understanding of vision therapy: Meir Schneider, Grace Hallaron and Peter Mansfield.

I would like to thank those who worked on the manuscript: Christine Kondrot, Shiva Pourazima, Bill Coors, Dahlia Hirsch, Roger Morrison, and Eileen Nauman provided much-needed encouragement by reviewing the entire manuscript prior to publication. In addition I would like to thank my secretary Cathie Youngans for her dedication and for her ability to keep me organized. And to Joanne Lew, for her illustrations, my appreciation.

I extend the deepest thanks to Gloria St John for her major contribution in producing this book. Her vast understanding of natural medicine contributed enormously to the final shape of this work. I am still in awe of her ability to not only grasp the essence of a subject, but render it into compelling prose in very short order. Her dedication to this project allowed me to produce this book in nearly record time.

Last I would like to thank all my patients for letting me be a partner in helping them improve their eyesight.

Edward Kondrot, MD

Contents

Foreword by William Coors
President, Coors Brewing

The scene is an ophthalmologist's office. The doctor is talking to a patient. "You have age-related macular degeneration. We call it ARMD. It is the leading cause of blindness in older people. We have no treatment for it. Come back and see me in three months." The patient wonders to himself, "Why?" This depressing news is given to thousands of people each year—people who visited the eye doctor because of recent changes they noticed in their vision.

I, too, heard these fateful words fifteen years ago. They were similar to the words I heard from my internist at Mayo Clinic some fifty years ago. My ailment at that time was an extreme case of 'executive burnout' which was not recognized by medical orthodoxy of that time. My internist's message had two parts. "We have good news and bad news for you. The good news is we can find nothing wrong with you. The bad news is we can do nothing for you."

Messages like these leave people with two choices— retire to a cave for the rest of your life or seek help elsewhere. Choosing the second alternative leads one into the vast and complex field of alternative (or what many now call complementary) medicine. For me, this was a long and frustrating journey, but it solved my problems.

It was only natural to pursue the same course when I received my ARMD diagnosis. Anyway you slice it, aging itself is a degenerative process that gets us all in the end. And the end will come when the first essential body part wears out beyond repair. ARMD is nothing more, or less, than the accelerated aging of an almost essential body part— the macula.

The human body is a remarkable aggregation of billions of individual cells, each one essential to the well being of the whole. Each cell requires a constant supply of nutrients, some highly specialized, to function properly. In addition, there must be an effective distribution system to carry the nutrients to every cell. The cells that comprise the cones and rods of the macula are no exception. Failure to provide the body with all its essential nutrients, or any impairment in the delivery system to the cells causes degeneration of the affected cells.

Equally important is the fact that the human body possesses the ability to repair itself provided it receives the tools and materials necessary for the repair job. One essential tool is mental attitude. We hear much about the healing power of prayer and the mind/body effect these days. The placebo effect is an example of the mind's encouraging the body to heal. And death by voodoo proves that the mind can destroy the body as well.

In my fifteen year battle with ARMD, I have concentrated on cardiovascular health, nutritional supplementation, immune system reinforcement, and mental attitude. I have lost ground in my left eye, but my right eye appears to be holding. As I write this text, I can see the letters perfectly. I don't see ARMD as curable, but I know for certain that its progress can be delayed. Perhaps, if caught early enough, it can be arrested.

Every single curative concept that I have heard of and used on myself is delineated in Dr. Kondrot's book. In addition, his book has alerted me to two previously unknown therapies. I plan to add homeopathy and microcurrent stimulation to my regimen.

At this writing I have sixteen more years of life expectancy. I have every confidence that at the end of those years, I will see well enough to enjoy a gorgeous sunset and feast on the faces of those I love. I can't urge you strongly enough to take the message of this book to heart. Neither Dr. Kondrot nor I can make you any promises, but there is one thing I can all but guarantee. You will see better longer, and you may even see well for the rest of your life.

Foreword by Dahlia Hirsch MD

Macular Degeneration can be a frightening word, and a frightening diagnosis, but it has come a long way. Twenty years ago, it was called Senile Macular Degeneration- a witness to the fact that doctors neither understood its development nor had much sensitivity to the human side of practicing medicine. Unfortunately many physicians still tell patients with this diagnosis that there is no therapy available to help them. This just isn't so. There are so many ways people can be helped, if we take the time to look at the individual and heal them as a whole person: mind, body, and spirit. Healing is the experience of "wholeness" and that means much more than what a person can read on a chart, which we artificially deem 'perfect vision'.

Similarly, the art of medicine means much more that giving a pill or performing surgery to achieve this socially defined goal of seeing well. As it turns out, there are many aspects of seeing: reading a chart, side or peripheral vision, color vision, contrast (shades of black, white, and gray), depth perception, brightness, interpretation of what is noticed, the response to it, and inner vision. A deficiency in one can often be compensated for by another. For instance in order to catch a ball most people need depth perception. However there was a great football player who had only one eye, and therefore no depth perception. He used other visual clues such as shadow and size of objects to catch the football very well.

The art of medicine is in guiding people to experience their highest potential in the safest way possible. In order to do this we must educate people and empower them to make choices and to know that all healing is possible. Without hope, no miracles can ever occur. Without inner vision, no new therapies can evolve. I remember when we removed cataracts under general anesthesia, and kept the patient in the hospital for two weeks. At every new discovery, there were the doubters, and they were loud and convincing. Eventually cataracts were removed in minutes with no stitches or hospital stays. I believe eventually we will prevent cataracts. It requires first that someone have the idea, or the vision, and then methods will follow. There will always be the doubters and the resisters, but without trying we will never know. The same is true for Macular Degeneration.

The evidence that antioxidants help prevent aging was presented over 20 years ago, and yet many doctors today have not shared that information with their patients. In a survey of cardiologists, 47% personally take antioxidants, but most don't discuss these supplements with their patients. This is unacceptable. We must teach patients about nutrition and supplements. Years ago doctors said stroke patients could not regain function, and therefore they were given no therapy. Not surprisingly, they didn't regain function. Someone had to change their mind—have a vision—and we now know that by working with the undamaged surrounding tissue people often regain much function after strokes.

We have good reason to believe that macular degeneration may be undergoing the same revolutionary changes. New ideas are being looked at, and some of them are translated into therapies that may work for many people. There are new surgical techniques and pharmaceutical drugs with great possibilities and often great risk. Other approaches are very safe and can be done at home by patients. I think it is imperative that macular degeneration patients be informed of these possibilities, and choose for themselves.

Finally, someone in the medical profession has stood up to share this information so that patients can choose. We cannot afford to do nothing while there are safe alternatives that have helped many people. Good nutrition is imperative to good sight. Good psychological well-being produces molecules of healing and is essential for good sight. Good air and breath and circulation are important. An active mind is important to receive and interpret images. It makes sense that if we believe exercise is good for the body, that it is also good for the eye, and that there might be special exercises for the eye that are also good for the body.

Educating patients takes hours of a doctor's time, and most doctors have not studied these ideas at all. Therefore it is imperative that patients educate themselves. But in this world of confusing information and misinformation, there is the dilemma of credibility. Whom can you trust? I commend Dr. Kondrot, a board certified and very busy and successful ophthalmologist, for taking the initiative and time to share a broad spectrum of discoveries with you in this book. The information is organized, factual, and simple yet thoroughly explained. The result is a very practical guide that anyone can use to evaluate choices and initiate a reasonable program for themselves. Every ophthalmologist should be grateful to Dr. Kondrot for answering the questions their patients ask. Hopefully they will recommend this book to their sight-challenged patients.

Dahlia Hirsch MD
Bel Air, Maryland

Introduction

I became a doctor because I wanted to help people and to heal people. Twenty-five years ago when I entered medical school, this was my goal. Today helping people to heal is still my goal, but the way I go about it is the result of a long personal and professional journey. When I graduated from Hahnemann Medical School in Philadelphia in 1977, I thought that I had everything I needed to accomplish my goal. Little did I know that the very name of my medical school foretold the path that awaited me.

I decided to specialize in diseases of the eye because it seemed that the most exciting research and advances in medicine and surgery were happening in that field. I very much wanted to contribute and see diseases that produce blindness and near blindness eliminated in my lifetime. I really believed it could happen; yet, after more than ten years of practice, I was far from being satisfied with my work. Most of my patients did not get better, and my treatments just delayed the inevitable worsening of their diseases. I began to ask myself if there was a better way.

I have always been competitive and liked to engage in very demanding and rigorous sports. While training for the Hawaii Ironman Triathlon in 1988, a friend suggested that I take a homeopathic remedy to help me cope with the muscle and joint pain of over-training. I was astonished at the results. My pain disappeared in a very short time, and there were no side effects from the remedy as there would have been if I had taken a prescription or an over-the-counter pain reliever. Being a scientist, I could not ignore what had happened to me, and I began to learn more about homeopathy.

My early study of homeopathy was limited to books. Soon I discovered a world of experts and lectures where my learning could expand rapidly. Along the way I heard about the Hahnemann College of Homeopathy, located near San Francisco. Could it be that I was destined to attend yet another school named after the founder of homeopathy, Samuel Hahnemann? I was, and for the next four years, traveled one long weekend each month to the Bay Area to study homeopathy. At first I thought it would be a breeze, given my many years of medical study. However, I found that homeopathy, like all complete systems of healing, was a very complex subject. I immersed myself in it, and now consider it the most rewarding thing I have undertaken in my life. When it came time for me to write my thesis in homeopathy, I decided to research how the early homeopaths treated eye disease in the 18th and 19th century. Because many of the old books have been preserved, I was able to uncover a wealth of information.

One of the things I learned about homeopathy is that many of the present masters of this medical art live and work in other countries. Homeopathy is very popular in England and other parts of Europe as well as in India. It was in India that I discovered three physicians who were able to teach me so much about using homeopathy to treat eye conditions. I made three trips to India, and each was unique and very meaningful to me. I was able to sit and observe the work of three leading homeopaths: Dr. Ramakrishnan of Madras, Dr Jugal Kishore in New Delhi, and Dr. K. P. Muzumdar in Bombay. Dr. Ramakrishnan, who specializes in the treatment of cancer with homeopathy, has become a close friend. He has also visited my office in Pittsburgh to consult with me on eye problem cases.

During this time, I also traveled to Germany as well as to many parts of the United States to attend seminars and learn all I could about the rich and evolving world of natural therapies for eye disease. I am very grateful to all my mentors and for this opportunity. It enriched me personally and allowed me to feel like the healer I always wanted to be.

The character of my practice began to change. Now I could offer hope to my patients with macular degeneration, diabetic retinopathy, glaucoma, cataract and eye strain. Furthermore, they could take charge of their illness and begin to heal by making lifestyle changes as well as by using natural healing techniques. Introducing homeopathy, along with nutrition and other natural methods of healing into my practice has vastly increased my satisfaction in being a doctor. It has also brought hope and relief to many of my patients. My enthusiasm for treating eye disease with a combination of natural treatments and conventional medicine prompted me to write this book. This is the first in a series of books dealing with the various eye conditions that respond to natural methods. These include Age-Related Macular Degeneration (ARMD), glaucoma, cataract, and eyestrain.

The subject of this book is macular degeneration, specifically, Age-Related Macular Degeneration (ARMD). Most people who have this disease are so fearful when they hear the diagnosis that they do not even understand what the condition or how they developed it. Most distressing of all, they have virtually no information about how to help themselves. Their doctors probably told them that nothing can be done for them, nothing can significantly retard or reverse their disease. If you or a loved one have been told that, *do not believe it.* Do not give up. Read this book and make the decision to implement these twelve steps as a way to begin taking control of your health and vision. Every one of these suggestions will benefit your overall health as well as improve your outlook and ability to cope. In addition to nutrition, herbs, and homeopathy, this book will describe microcurrent stimulation and chelation. These two therapies have produced dramatic results in my patients with macular degeneration. Explore with me these exciting alternatives that can bring back your sight!

This book deals only with alternative treatments for Age-Related Macular Degeneration. These include some that are now being studied within conventional medicine as well as those that focus either on lifestyle change or treatments that have not yet been proven to be effective in scientific research. While trying these approaches, you should remain under the care of your ophthalmologist and have your vision checked periodically. He or she may recommend other treatments, some of which may not be available at the time of this writing. If this is the case, you need to evaluate these options. Fortunately, most of the recommendations in this book complement conventional treatment. Your sight is precious, and you need to feel assured that you are doing everything possible to maintain it.

Edward Kondrot MD
Pittsburgh, PA
www.homeopathiceye.com

Step 1 | Know Your Condition

Chances are, you are reading this because you or a dear one has been told that he or she has Macular Degeneration. Your first challenge was to become accustomed to the name of this disorder, which is also called Age-Related Macular Degeneration, or ARMD. Anyway you think about it, it is not friendly. 'Macular' is probably a strange term to you and 'degeneration' does not sound like something moving in the right direction! Adding to your confusion is the fact that your doctor may not have spent much time discussing this with you. There are several reasons why eye doctors tend to be very brief when people are diagnosed with this condition. Macular Degeneration (ARMD) affects parts of the eye that are unfamiliar to most people. Launching into an explanation of the anatomy of the eye as well as telling someone they have a serious disease is more than many doctors want to do at one time. In addition, you were probably too stunned to take in new information. I can tell you this, no doctor likes to give this diagnosis to a person because the doctor knows that the patient will be apprehensive and fearful—and with good reason since conventional medicine has very little to offer people with ARMD. Your doctor has most likely told you to go home and look at a grid (See Resources section for the Amsler

Know Your Condition

Grid) on a piece of cardboard every day and call him if things change dramatically. If you asked him whether there was anything that could be done, he may have told you to take some vitamins with zinc as a supplement. Perhaps his lack of enthusiasm made you feel that this would not help much.

You Will not Lose All your Sight!

So here you are, looking at the Amsler Grid faithfully and wondering how soon you will go blind and becoming more and more depressed. Let's start with the good news. *You will not go completely blind from ARMD – ever.* This condition results in the loss of central vision only, and the degree of vision lost varies greatly. Even those who do nothing to help their bodies cope with ARMD, and will not lose all their sight. If you read this book and make a sincere effort to implement its twelve steps, you have an excellent change of retaining your current level of vision and even restoring some of what you have lost. Believe me. I have seen it happen with my patients. You have been told nothing else can be done. This is not true! Something can be done, and I am very happy to share my experiences with you. The Twelve Steps to Better Eyesight can improve your vision!

> James Buchman, one of my patients who has Stargardt Macular Degeneration, was told by his former doctor to go home and wait for blindness to set in— and to be grateful that it might take five years. His wife Robin writes: "James could not believe that he might not be able to see our children grow, watch sunsets, enjoy paintings, and, still more

frightening, lose his job as a teacher, jeopardizing the family's economic situation. I searched the internet and finally found out about your practice, Dr. Kondrot, and Microcurrent Stimulation. We thank you for giving us hope. Perhaps James will now be able to see his children grow, maintain an active sight-filled life, and pursue his career desires. Without your help we would be preparing for a seeing-eye dog, Braille, and similar life changes."

"Dr. Kondrot...Your continuing quest to seek answers when others have quit has changed my son's life...."

Ken Johnson writes this about his son David, another of my patients: "Two and one half months after receiving Microcurrent Stimulation (MCS) at your office, David... is signing up for college courses. He is talking about driving. Your continuing quest to seek answers when others have quit has changed my son's life. He is now hopeful and optimistic. He is safer and life is easier for him. My wife and I cannot thank you enough.

Know Your Condition

Who Develops Age-Related Macular Degeneration?

Macular Degeneration affects 13 million Americans. Most of them are over the age of 65, but certain hereditary conditions may cause it to develop in younger individuals. Those of you reading this book who have congenital macular degeneration, please be reassured that these methods will also work in your situation. In fact, younger people often respond beautifully to many of these treatments. Persons over the age of 75 have a 30% chance of developing ARMD; it rarely affects anyone younger than 55 years old. Caucasians develop it more than persons of color because they have less pigment in their retina, especially if they have blue, grey, or green eyes. It affects men and women equally. People who are nearsighted (myopic) have a greater chance of developing this condition as do people who work or spend a lot of time out of doors and are exposed to ultraviolet radiation from sunlight.

What Causes ARMD?

Doctors like to say that we don't know what causes ARMD. However, when you look at the relationship between age and the onset of ARMD, I bet you can guess that the same things which cause so many of the afflictions of the elderly are somehow linked to ARMD. These afflictions are arthritis, diabetes, hypertension, atherosclerosis, obesity and high cholesterol. Much as we don't like to admit it, most of these other conditions result from our lifestyle—poor diet, lack of exercise, and the inability to cope with stress. The good news is that things that are caused by factors we can identify are more likely to improve when we eliminate those factors. Actually, I

10

believe every disease and disorder has a cause, even child-hood cancers and all sorts of things medical science likes to say cannot be explained. The truth is they cannot be explained within the framework of their thinking and understanding. Not too long ago, doctors scoffed at the idea that diet had anything to do with heart disease. Until Dr. Dean Ornish proved, within the framework of scientific research, that an improved diet, and a program of exercise, and social support along with relaxation help reverse physical degeneration, it was impossible to convince doctors of this link. Now that it has been established, the medical community has accepted this idea, and lifestyle recommendations are the norm, not just for people with heart disease, but for everyone. We all know that eating less fat and sugar and exercising more are good for us. Coincidentally, these same recommendations have been shown to help with diabetes, arthritis, and all the other chronic degenerative conditions that affect our aging population. There is that word again — degenerative.

What Is Degeneration?

Generation means that something new or fresh is being born. Degeneration means that something is dying or passing away. When used to describe something in the body, degeneration means a gradual breaking down of tissues or organs, resulting in reduced function of the parts affected. Degeneration from arthritis means that the affected joint does not work as well as it did before it degenerated. In Macular Degeneration the eyes do not work as well as they once did. Specifically, vision in the center of the visual field gets fainter and fainter until finally there is hardly any way to see things straight on.

The fact that this is a slow process, that it affects older persons, and that it continues to get worse if nothing is done to change the person's lifestyle, leads me to believe firmly that the same factors that produce all degenerative changes in the body are involved in ARMD. Studies have shown that there is a higher incidence of ARMD in persons who have hypertension, diabetes, and conditions which cause clogging or hardening of the arteries. Therefore, if we can halt or reverse the damage done to our blood vessels and joints through adopting a healthier lifestyle, we can expect improvement in eye conditions like ARMD. This is not just theory; I have seen it work with my patients and so have a number of other ophthalmologists. An added bonus is that the lifestyle recommendations for ARMD are bound to improve other degenerative conditions that patients may have.

I want you to understand ARMD, not only in terms of the physical changes in the eye, but as a disease of lifestyle and aging with *symptoms* affecting the eye. Take a moment to honestly assess your overall health in terms of the dietary and exercise recommendations that we all know about already. We all know we should eat five to six servings of vegetables and fruit daily, exercise aerobically several times a week, and use some form of focused relaxation technique daily. It goes without saying that smoking at all and alcohol to excess are taboo. Ditto for sugar and fat from meat and dairy products. How do you rate? Do you think there might actually be a cause for the degenerative condition that has affected your eyes? If so, are you willing to try to eliminate the cause and adopt techniques and healing methods that might restore your vision? I hope so, for your sake. What have you got to lose? Please begin to implement these recommendations today!

Know Your Specific Diagnosis

When your doctor gave you the news about ARMD, he probably told you that you have either 'dry' or 'wet' ARMD. This has nothing to do with how dry or teary your eyes feel to you. It refers rather to two completely different reasons why the macula in your eye or eyes has begun to degenerate. By the way, you may have ARMD in only one eye, or you may have Dry ARMD in one eye and Wet ARMD in the other. If so, the chances of it affecting the other eye are quite high, unfortunately. Going back to the wet and dry terms, 'wet' ARMD occurs when the blood vessels in the back of the eye begin to leak fluid or blood in the back portion of your inner eye. It affects 10% of persons with ARMD. Dry ARMD, which affects 90% of persons with ARMD results from a buildup of cellular waste products in the back part of the inner eye. It is very important that you know which type you have. If you have forgotten, or your doctor neglected to tell you, pick up the phone and call him or her to find out. This is a first step in empowering yourself to get better.

Wet Macular Degeneration has certain characteristics and prognosis (expected outcome). I have observed that some cases of Wet ARMD come on suddenly after a period of stress or shock, and a person may lose a great deal of vision in a short period of time. One of the treatments for wet ARMD uses laser surgery to cauterize the leaky blood vessels. This measure may preserve more vision in the long run, but usually results in worse vision in the short run because healthy tissue is almost always destroyed along with the diseased vessels. Wet ARMD progresses faster than Dry ARMD and may result in greater loss of vision over a shorter time period. Wet ARMD is actually quite distinct from Dry ARMD and will respond to different alternative medical treatments than the dry type.

Dry ARMD results from an accumulation of dead cells in the area in the back of the inner eyeball where the retina and macula are located. The macula is actually the center of the retina. That is why, even when it degenerates, you can still see peripherally, or images made on the outer circle of the retina. As dead cells build up on the macula, they do two things: they block the macula's ability to produce images and, they corrode this delicate tissue, leading to permanent degeneration. It is not understood exactly why the dead cells begin to build up and the 'clean up' mechanism that worked for sixty or more years starts to malfunction. That is, it is not clear from a molecular scientific understanding. But you already know that I have some strong suspicions that this process is what we call aging. This means that metabolic waste products begin to clog our system and new cells do not regenerate quickly enough to cope with this detritus. The reason this affects the macula so profoundly is that this is a very small, highly sensitive area, an area that is prone to accumulate waste by virtue of its high metabolic needs. The macula requires more oxygen, nutrients, and energy compared to other areas of the body. Therefore, early signs of more generalized degenerative changes may appear first in this area.

Symptoms of Macular Degeneration

If you know you have Macular Degeneration, you are familiar with the vision changes that prompted you to visit an ophthalmologist and get tested and diagnosed. If you have experienced changes in your vision and may be wondering whether you have ARMD, I will briefly describe its early symptoms. Of course, other eye conditions may have these same symptoms, so it is a good idea to be checked by a qualified eye care professional as soon as you are aware of them.

The first thing most people notice is a lessening of their sight as they look straight at things, like print, faces or clocks. This may be a dimming, a blurring, or actual 'holes' or black spots in the vision. Extreme light sensitivity and poor night vision also precede ARMD in many cases. Light-to-dark adaptation, needed when you try to find a seat in a movie theatre, is apt to be very slow. Because doctors do not think that anything can be done to halt the progress of this disease, the public has not been educated to be aware of these early symptoms. However, I believe that if people who notice any of these changes in their vision begin a program like the one described in the following chapters, they may be able to arrest the damage to their eyes and maintain near normal vision. ARMD, like most degenerative processes, takes a long time to develop. People may feel that it came on suddenly, but that is because one day they were fine and the next day they received a diagnosis where they feared they may go blind. It does not happen that way. Anyone over 35 years old who is reading this book should take some of the steps toward better eye health. Those who have been diagnosed with ARMD should take them all.

There Is Hope

Once you understand the degenerative aspect of Macular Degeneration you can design a strategy to halt the degeneration and reverse the damage it has already done. Studies in aging have identified several key components that you must include in your strategy. I have listed them below, and use them throughout the book as we discuss specific measures to reverse ARMD.

In this book, I am going to talk about diet, vitamin and mineral supplements, homeopathy, relaxation, exercises for the eye and whole body, and some techniques that may be new to you—chelation and microcurrent stimulation. While these may seem to be very distinct approaches to health, all of these involve the four key components of anti-aging.

---

1. Increase oxygenation of tissues

2. Make the metabolic processes more efficient

3. Target nourishment to tissues and cells

4. Detoxify tissues and cells

A program that incorporates these objectives will certainly enhance your overall health. Although, I am not an advocate of living to over 100 years, I am a firm believer in the quality of life and I want the same for my patients. Our world needs vigorous elders. Medical science can keep us alive longer, but only by taking responsibility for their health can individuals make that extra time useful and enjoyable.

Though we are just in the first chapter, you have probably already encountered some ideas that you will not see in other books on Macular Degeneration. One idea is that how you live probably has something to do with your developing this condition. Some people feel blamed by this. A better way to look at it is that if you had something to do with getting ARMD, you may be able to do something about it.

Heal Your Eyes, Heal Your Self

I want to emphasize now, at the beginning, that every step you take moves you closer to the next step by actually making you healthier. When you are healthier, you will feel stronger. Even though you have a serious condition, you do not have to tackle everything at once. The slow and steady approach will work wonders for you! Try to work on several fronts at one time, however. For example, even though you may be a beginner at improving your diet, read ahead to the chapters on treatment ideas and begin to implement at least one of them. This book offers three major ways you can help yourself and protect your vision. You can start working on all of them simultaneously. They are:

Lifestyle Modification
- Diet
- Exercise
- Stress Management

Self Care
- Supplements
- Eye Nutrients
- Herbs
- Eye Exercises

Treatment
- Homeopathy
- Chelaton
- Microcurrent Stimulation

Know Your Condition

Hopefully, you feel motivated, not overwhelmed, at this point. Remember, you have already taken the first step, and are about to take the next.

One very important step you can take to empower yourself right now is to share this book with a friend or family member. Choose someone who will support you in taking charge of your health in general and your eye health in particular. You may enounter resistance from those who do not believe in the power of self care or who have not heard of the options we will explore in this book. It is only human to experience self doubt when naysayers are all around! This is where your support person comes in. He or she can keep you on track and motivated as you continue to take steps to heal your vision.

Checklist for Step One

√   Know your diagnosis

√   Use the Amsler Grid

√   Identify other health problems

√   Select a support person

Know Your Condition

Step 2 | Feast Your Eyes

A beautiful scene or picture is known as a feast for the eyes because what is taken in, or viewed, is considered nourishing in some sense. It may seem like a strange idea, but certain foods are also a feast for the eyes. Experts in nutrition have long known that certain organs and tissues of the body respond to specific types of food. These organ-specific foods contain nutrients that are needed in abundance by the targeted part of the body. Carrots and spinach, as we all have learned, are said to be good for the eyes because they contain an abundance of Vitamin A. Unfortunately, most of us are not very sophisticated about nutrition. We may not have learned much more than that about nutrition for the eyes. As it turns out, there are many other foods that are good for the eyes.

In this chapter we are going to talk about planning and adopting a diet that can not only preserve sight but may restore it for those who have already developed Age-Related Macular Degeneration (ARMD). Some of the dietary suggestions may not appeal to you at first. Perhaps recalling our discussion in Chapter One will help you overcome your reluctance to change. There I suggested that if something about your lifestyle allowed you to develop ARMD, then there is a good chance that something could be changed in your lifestyle to promote healing not just your ARMD but the underlying conditions that led to its development. Your diet is a good place to start.

> Dr. Dahlia Hirsch is an ophthalmologist who practices holistic medicine in Maryland. She has helped a number of patients with ARMD change their diets along the guidelines we will suggest in this chapter. She says, "In ten years of practice, I can say that those patients who eat this way and take vitamins and supplements almost invariably tell me that they are seeing better."

At birth, our bodies are composed of tissues and organs made from the nutrients in the food our mother consumed during pregnancy. After that, we are pretty much self-made in that what we eat produces the energy to grow and maintain our bodies. Few of us enjoy a lifetime of optimal nutrition. The result is that, as we age, our bodies lose their ability to cope with the stressors of life. By stressors I mean the exposure to sunlight, pollution, poor quality water, and a host of other factors that make up modern life. As we age, past dietary 'sins' (remember all those hamburgers and fries consumed during your teens) begin to take their toll. Chronic and degenerative disease may set in. In addition, older bodies have the burden of maintaining health and strength in the face of the metabolic slowdown that accounts for the natural process of aging. We can't fight that. What we can do, however, to provide ourselves with optimum nutrition in order to minimize the impact of this aging process. If you have ARMD, you face the double challenge of trying to arrest or reverse it while continuing to maintain health and strength. This situation calls for a focused program of nutrition with an emphasis on wholesome food as well as supplements. Supplements are just what they are called. They do not substitute for good food. They add to a diet that is already rich and nourishing. I will talk about your supplement needs in a later chapter. Now for the diet.

Food As Medicine

A person who has developed a degenerative disease needs to start thinking of food as medicine, in fact the very best medicine. The more you can meet your nutritional needs from food the better. Our bodies are built to digest and utilize food. Nutrients in capsules and tablets are second best and only needed when our need for nutrients is so great that it cannot be met by diet alone. People with ARMD fall into this category, and you will need to supplement your diet. However, the dietary program I am going to recommend can be considered baseline nutrition for the rest of your life. There is a bonus as I have already indicated. Nature, in her wisdom, determined that whatever is good for your eyes is good for the rest of you also. So, those with hypertension, arthritis, obesity, hypothyroidism, diabetes, and coronary artery disease will find that these conditions also improve on "the feast for the eyes" diet.

> Dr. Hirsch has noticed that a large number of people with ARMD have another serious degenerative disease. "Either these diseases are similar, or one

> causes the other, or the medication pre-
> scribed for chronic degenerative condi-
> tions plays a role in the development of
> ARMD. Some of the medications deplete
> vitamins and minerals, especially zinc."

Another important reason to consider food as medicine when you have ARMD is that there is no other medicine available. There are conventional treatments for the
condition which include laser surgery for the wet type,
and radiation. There are many natural techniques such as
eye exercises, chelation, homeopathy, and microcurrent
stimulation, which we will discuss and recommend later
in this book. There are no drugs; there is no medicine
for ARMD. Therefore it makes sense to consider food
as your first medicine. If your diet is good, all the other
techniques you use to help your condition will work more
effectively. Your daily nutrition is like your checking account. Although you make deposits and withdrawals,
hopefully the balance is always sufficient to cover your
checks. Then, when there is a surplus, you can open a
savings account. You hold this money in reserve until
you need extra funds (or nutritional support) to cover
an emergency. Finally, you secure your future with funds
in the money market or stocks. Using a technique like
homeopathy or microcurrent stimulation or chelation,
when you are not adequately nourished on a daily basis,
is like using your money market funds to meet the ex-
penses of daily living. It is simply not the proper use of
a resource.

Add in order to Subtract

Due to the research findings that show how poor diet contributes to chronic diseases, most of us have a working knowledge of the proper diet. It is all about eliminating the things that we love and that taste best to us. Forget about fat, butter, eggs, whole milk, soft drinks, beer, cookies, ice cream, red meat. Right? Wrong. That is, at best, part of the picture. A proper diet means eating high quality, non-toxic, nutritious food. And that can include any of the items listed above when taken in moderation. The problem with the Standard American Diet (SAD) is that people try to eliminate the foods that are bad for them, like those listed above, but they have no idea how to include the foods that are good for them. Most people are quite unfamiliar with good food. Think about it. The middle-aged or older person of today, the one most likely to have ARMD, grew up in an era where commercially prepared, chemically-laced food was considered good. In this era, vegetables meant frozen peas; fish sticks were considered a good source of protein; cookies came in a box full of preservatives and partially hydrogenated oils; eating out meant fast food and cola. For most people on a SAD, eggs, butter, and whole milk are as close as they get to real food! Naturally, they don't want to give them up.

I am going to suggest that you start thinking about what to add to your diet and forget, for the time being, about what to eliminate. I am using this approach because I trust your body. I trust it to respond to real, whole food and begin to crave it. And when you crave it, you will eat more of it, and then you will not be so hungry for bad food. Sound too simple? Well, think about how far you have come with the elimination or subtraction plan. Perhaps you have substituted margarine for butter and powdered egg whites for eggs, and non-fat milk for milk. Do you enjoy these foods? Probably not. Are they good for you? Not especially. So, let's explore another approach.

The author of a very useful and popular book on healthful cooking, *Laurel's Kitchen*, says that the first problem with becoming a vegetarian is learning how to fill in the hole on the plate left by the absence of meat! The same thing can be said about making the shift to a nutritious, non-toxic diet, that is a feast for the eyes to boot! What in the world do you put on your plate in place of all your old favorites? How often have you read about the importance of eating whole grains, nuts, legumes, fruits, and vegetables and had your mind glaze over? You may have said something to yourself like, "I've got a box of brown rice in the cupboard." Do you feel you really know what real, whole food is? Can you cook with it? Do you know where to find it? Clue: It is not in the supermarket. In the supermarket, you will find food that is the product of the food industry—the highly lucrative business of producing food. This includes the heavy use of pesticides, herbicides, chemical fertilizer, preservatives, stray genes, and anything else that will keep the cost of production low and the shelf life (profit) as high as possible.

Farmers' Markets

Before we begin talking about what to eat, let's find out where is the real food. We'll begin with produce. The very best place to find real produce is at a Farmers' Market. Many communities have these, and the really fortunate ones have a market where a number of growers sell organic produce. Organic simply means that the produce had no chemical pesticides, fertilizers, or sprays used during the growing cycle of the food. A step down from true organic is the use of pesticide sprays on mature fruit and vegetables. Farmers who do this usually have a sign indicating that they use them. Sprays can be washed off before the food is eaten, unlike commercial fertilizers and pesticides that are taken up by the roots and absorbed by the leaves, becoming an integral part of the plant.

As a first step to improve your diet, locate a Farmers' Market near you and visit it. Allow yourself to wander around until you get familiar. (It is considered good to bring your own basket or marketing bag to reduce the use of plastic.) While you are looking around, feeling confused about kohlrabi and Chinese eggplant, take a look at the organic farmers themselves. You'll see how healthy they look. They eat a lot of this stuff. They are also eager to talk about all the strange things they grow and will be happy to advise you in matters of preparation.

On your first trip, purchase some collard greens, spinach, or kale. These three vegetables have been proven to provide the form of Vitamin A most easily used by the eyes. Buy some apples and other familiar items on your first trip, too. With some greens in the fridge and a bowl of apples on the table, you are off to a good start in changing your diet. For the first week, eat some of these greens in place of the frozen peas and anemic lettuce you might be accustomed to eating; eat the apples whenever you want to snack. Plan to visit the Farmers' Market regularly and buy one new vegetable each week. By the way, unlike the supermarket, Farmers' Markets have only seasonal items, so you may see a pile of beans one week but none the next. In this way, you will become accustomed to a wide variety of produce.

Feast Your Eyes

A word about quantity. When you ate those frozen peas, you probably had a small pile of them in a corner of your plate. That is not enough—even for frozen peas. Start eating larger servings of vegetables. Prepare them as side dishes. Serve fruit for dessert. Eat salad with everything. Try this for a dinner: a large baked potato, one-half baked squash, a large portion of collard greens, salad with seasonal raw vegetables, corn bread, and watermelon for dessert. Go ahead and use a little butter! The idea is to fill up on good stuff, so you will not be so hungry for empty calories.

Health Food Stores

The next place to look for real food is in a health food store. Go on a prospecting trip first if it seems intimidating. Maybe one of your relatives or neighbors is a health nut. Ask them to take you to their favorite store. Remember, we're not buying supplements yet, just food, so you can focus on food alone. The produce in a health food store will offer more variety than that at the Farmers' Market. You will find some tasty out-of-season items to add to your menus. You may need to shop for most of your produce in the health food store if you do not have a Farmers' Market in your community or when the market is not in session (wintertime). Health food store produce will be more expensive than the produce you formerly bought in the supermarket. Forget about making comparisons. You can only compare price; you cannot compare the quality. If you have ARMD or any other degenerative disease, you need to spend money on good food. Your savings will come when you stop buying junk food. Right now, though, we are adding, not eliminating.

During your first visit to the health food store, plan to buy grains, nuts, and legumes. Sound squirrelly? Again, we are going to keep it simple. Buy some organic, short grain brown rice out of a bin (not a box). You know what brown rice is. You can take a peek at the quinoa (pronounced keenwa) and the millet, but you don't have to venture that far yet. Then buy some almonds. No, they are not slivered and in plastic. They are whole and in the bins, too. Take them home and roast them in an iron skillet or toast them in the oven until they start to pop. Let them cool. Eat them when you are hungry for a snack. Get some pumpkin seeds and toast them in the oven too. Grain, nut, legume! You are all set to add them to your greens and apples. If you like eggs, you might be pleased to know that those laid by hens raised on a natural diet without hormones, antibiotics, or pesticide-laden food have been proven to have less cholesterol than commercial eggs. There is no advantage to eating fertile eggs, but get them if you wish. You will probably see a whole host of other organic dairy selections—milk, butter, and cheese. Use your discretion and try them if you have not been advised to curtail fat and cholesterol intake. Take a look at the yogurt. Fewer flavors and options will be offered, but you will get more digestion-enhancing cultures in the health food store brands.

Not everything in health food stores is particularly healthy. In trying to appeal to the American palate, they carry prepared food and imitation items like fake sausage made from soy products. None of these things will enhance your health particularly; but they will probably not harm you too much. My guess is that if you really love sausage, you will not like fake sausage. Just begin to fill up your plate and your stomach with whole food, and your craving for sausage will probably subside. Many health food stores carry high quality meat such as range-free chickens and pesticide-free fish. Feel free to add these to your diet if you wish.

Now that you know the way, shop at the Farmers' Market and the health food store until it becomes a habit. Experiment with a wide variety of food items. Learn or re-learn to cook or pay someone to do it for you. There is no way around this. You must prepare meals fresh and eat at home a great deal of the time. When you eat out, go to ethnic restaurants and have a good time. Do not eat at fast food restaurants. The fat, salt, and sugar content of their food may actually make you sick once you have feasted on real food for a while. By adding all these good things to your diet, you will naturally become more discriminating, and many of the things you formerly ate will lose their appeal.

Why Organic?

You may be wondering why I am so firm about your buying organic produce. The answer is that I assume you have or may be a candidate for ARMD, which, as we have already discussed, is a degenerative disease. Degeneration happens in the presence of certain conditions. One of them is having a toxic inner environment. All the toxins in your body get there because you admit them in some way. They come through the air you breathe, the water you drink, the food you eat. (By the way, get a good quality water filter on your next trip to the health food store.) In recommending the dietary changes in these pages, I am trying to help you detoxify your body. Why? I want it to be freed up to help you cope with life, aging, and healing your ARMD. There are more ways to detoxify. One of them is chelation therapy which I will explain in a later chapter. But the key to success and greater health is to reduce your toxic load on a daily basis. Therefore, my approach is two-pronged: stop adding to your toxic load by improving your diet, and eliminate the toxins you have accumulated through exercise and treatments like chelation therapy.

Eating organic produce eliminates the toxins contributed by farming chemicals. Eating whole foods eliminates the toxins contributed by chemical preservatives, additives, and artificial nutrients. By whole foods, I mean items that are as close to the way they grow as possible. A freshly caught fish might be quick frozen and be very close to its original state. Fish sticks are far from it! Brown rice has the nutrient rich hull still surrounding its kernel. You get the idea.

Change Like the Tortoise

Many books on regaining health have chapters on diet and nutrition. Usually they launch into a list of foods that you must eat as well as those you must avoid. After that, they give you pages and pages of recipes, most containing unfamiliar ingredients. This racing ahead and then stopping is like the way the hare ran the famous race against the tortoise. I am suggesting you take a lesson from the tortoise. Change slowly but steadily. Shop at the right places; become comfortable with many items at your new shopping locations; learn how to make a few good meals and snacks.

What to Add

Later in this book, I will tell you all about the supplements you will need to add to your good diet, and you will need to supplement. Remember, you are trying to arrest a degenerative condition or, if possible, reverse it. This requires a full-blown attempt to improve your nutritional status. We have all heard that carrots are good for the eyes, and they are. The thing that makes them good is the presence of beta carotene, the nutrient that converts to Vitamin A on an as-needed basis. Researchers have found, however, that other foods are an even richer source of beta carotene. The winners here are kale, spinach, and collard greens. You should still seek out orange, red, and yellow fruits and vegetables for their beta carotene, but do not let a day pass without at least one large serving of kale, spinach, or collard greens. Secondary choices for beta carotene are broccoli, Brussels sprouts, cabbage, cauliflower, pumpkin, fresh parsley, green peas, and raw tomato.

The next nutrient you need to obtain from food in a significant quantity is zinc. Sources of zinc are oysters, crabs, and bran cereals. Selenium is very important in eye health since it protects against ultraviolet light damage from sunlight. Selenium has been depleted from our soil, so a lot of the commercially-grown produce contributes very little of this mineral, even if the item is traditionally known to be high in selenium. Begin to add organic red chard, oats, brown rice, barley, wheat bran, nuts, and garlic along with orange juice to your diet.

All fats are not the same. While I strongly urge you to abandon margarine and limit saturated fats such as that found in meat and dairy products, it does not mean that you cannot have fat. On the contrary, the fats named Omega-3 and Omega-6 are vital for their role in lubricating delicate eye tissues and clearing clogged arteries. Food sources of these oils are salmon, sardines, tuna, and cod liver, flaxseed and olive oils. Add one large serving of at least one of these to your daily diet. You will find flaxseed oil in the refrigerated case at your health food store. Keep it refrigerated at home, too. Eat two tablespoons daily or use it as a dressing on salads.

One of the newer diet ideas I'm recommending is replacing some of the carbohydrates in your diet with protein. As a nation, we have become overloaded with carbohydrates. The concern about fat in meat and dairy products has produced a real carbohydrate craze. We have been told to eat pasta, salad, cereal, and bread. We have been advised not to eat fatty meat or full fat dairy products in the dietary gospel of the past decades. However, some new research, particularly, in the realm of obesity, has caused a partial retraction of that gospel. I find the work of Barry Sears, author of *The Zone* and *Mastering the Zone*, to be quite compelling. Other popular authors have built upon his core concept. The idea is that the production of insulin is related to weight gain, and insulin production soars when we overload on carbohydrates. Our dietary fads of the past decades may be to blame for the increased incidence of diabetes in adults. All that pasta and bread, even the whole grain products, have been quietly converted to fat by our bodies all these years.

Ideally, you should try to balance carbohydrates with protein and fat at each meal or snack. I urge you to take a look at one of these authors' books. You will probably find your thinking about nutrition modified considerably. One of the things I like about Sears' approach is his emphasis on vegetables and fruit for carbohydrates. When balancing a meal in terms of protein, carbohydrates, and fat, it makes sense to think about bountiful servings of spinach instead of a tiny bit of pasta on your plate as the carbohydrate allotment. The improved digestion and increased energy levels reported by many who have tried the zone approach, along with the filling and appetizing meals, make it worth trying. I hope you do so.

Feast Your Eyes

A word about preparation. Now that you know what to eat, be careful in your preparation. Yes to steaming or sauteing vegetables and poaching or grilling fish. Nix to frying or overcooking. You paid too much money for this food to ruin its value through poor cooking. High temperatures kill the nutrients in vegetables and cause oil to become carcinogenic.

Digestion

It has been found that many people who develop degenerative eye diseases also have poor digestion. In some cases digestion may be so severe that they have developed Crohn's disease or irritable bowel syndrome. In many cases, it simply means that the production of digestive enzymes by the liver and pancreas and hydrochloric acid by the stomach is sluggish. Feeling bloated, gaseous, or experiencing heartburn after eating are some of the signs of poor digestion. If you have these symptoms with any regularity, you need to support your digestion with enzyme supplements and hydrochloric acid. This will ensure that all those good nutrients become bio-available for your body to use and that they do not pass out as undigested waste. See the chapter on supplements for more complete information about this important step.

Dr. Hirsch has very wisely observed that three things are required to allow diet to work in a therapeutic way. "First, food must be grown in an appropriate way so that it has nutrients. Second, the person must be able to digest the food. Third, the food must be assimilated,

34

meaning that blood vessels are in good
shape to deliver nutrients to the cells."

I did not include recipes in this book because there are a lot of good recipe books around. Do buy one for yourself but make it a simple one. My approach to good nutrition is based on counseling many, many people. Most of them did not even cook for themselves. They ate out, got senior meals (most of these are lethal by the way), snacked endlessly, or opened cans. I realized that telling them to eat six to seven servings of produce a day was like telling them to begin speaking a foreign language. They had no idea how to go about making the needed changes in their diet. It seemed overwhelming and certainly not something they could take up in the face of a condition that limited their vision. That is why I broke it down into several easy steps. The idea is to keep at it and change underlying habits of shopping and meal preparation. Most of my patients were willing to do this when I explained that not only was food their best medicine, it was their only medicine. I hope you will feel this way too.

> Food is not only your best medicine,
> it is your only medicine.

Checklist for Step Two

√ Find a source for organic produce

√ Visit a health food store and make a purchase

√ Cook and eat a new vegetable each week for two months

√ Find a healthful cookbook you like

√ Increase low fat protein in your diet

√ Decrease carbohydrates

√ Reduce fat and sugar intake

√ Eliminate margarine and coffee from your diet

√ Improve your digestion

Step 3   Exercise

This chapter leads you to the next step in healing your vision problem – exercise. Exercise stimulates the repair mechanisms of the body. We are meant to move. Observe a small child if you have any doubts about this. They are virtually never still! In native settings, people move about until very late in life. Unfortunately our tendency to become immobile from aches, pains, and the loss of strength and stamina results primarily from our sedentary ways. In the previous chapter, I talked about how to keep your body parts nourished and lubricated. Now I will discuss how to keep them moving. If a car is not used for a month, the mechanical parts in the engine will begin to deteriorate. The same thing happens to your body. This chapter is about whole body exercise. The next chapter will talk about the specific exercises for the eyes.

In recent years, scientists have learned a great deal about exercise. As a result, virtually everybody believes that he/she should exercise. The problem is there are a lot of people, over 50 percent in fact, who do not exercise. If you are one of the people who exercised before you developed ARMD, then your challenge is to modify your program, if necessary, to cope with reduced vision. Perhaps you also need a little motivation and encouragement if you are feeling depressed and hopeless about the future. If you did not exercise regularly before developing ARMD, your challenge is to begin doing so at a time in life when you find many things more difficult. Although you may at first feel daunted by the idea of launching an exercise program now, exercise and movement can actually offer you more benefits than it offers a sighted person.

Why exercise?

There are many types of exercise, and we will discuss each type later in this chapter. The important thing to know is that any type—from aerobics to stretching—offers several key benefits to persons with low vision.

The first and most important benefit of exercise is its ability to combat depression. Movement increases the production of natural endorphins, the body's mood elevators. In one study, depressed people were assigned to one of three groups: those who exercised aerobically on a regular basis, those who took anti-depressants, and those who did both. The investigators predicted that those who both exercise and took anti-depressants would feel most relief from their depression. Everyone was surprised to learn that those who used exercise alone to combat depression reported feeling better than either of the other two groups after several weeks. It is quite normal to feel a low mood and depression after learning one has ARMD. However, exercise can provide a new focus for activity and actually change your biochemical state so significantly that depression can be overcome.

The second benefit of exercise is its ability to improve your confidence and sense of safety as you continue your normal activities with reduced vision. Fully sighted persons depend almost exclusively upon visual cues to guide them in moving about. One reason for this is that most modern people are out of touch with their bodies. Native people were and are able to move through completely black forests and jungles at night, relying on their senses of smell, hearing, and their kinesthetic sense. Kinesthetic means the sensation of bodily position, presence, or movement resulting chiefly from the stimulation of nerve endings in muscles, tendons, and joints. For example, you know that you are standing on the floor because the nerves in the soles of your feet are stimulated by contact with the floor. You know you have reached a wall when you bump into it. Many persons who lose some of their sight feel disoriented in space because they can no longer use visual cues and they have had little experience using their other senses. This disorientation causes them to lose their balance, feel clumsy, bump into things, and even get hurt. Exercise can restore a sense of confidence in your body. It can open up neural pathways and allow you to feel parts of your body that have had no sensation. The ability to feel your limbs and trunk will increase your sense of security in spatial orientation and allow you to move more gracefully and confidently. You will probably begin to feel a new relationship with your body once you realize how much you have lost contact with feeling it.

Grace Halloran is a woman who has pioneered a method of healing retinitis pigmentosa and other eye conditions, including ARMD. She suffered from the genetically transmitted condition from the time she was in her twenties. Determined not to lose all her sight, she defied all odds as well as the scientific community in designing a program to restore vision for those afflicted with this condition. In her autobiographical book, *Amazing Grace*, she tells the story of a time when her vision was low and she needed to walk outside in the forested area around her mountain home. Even as she panicked because she could not see, she realized that her bare feet could sense obstacles such as boulders and holes in the path. "I was determined to increase my overall awareness by using my feet. After all, feet are the primal contact with the earth, always receiving information. The signals, once interpreted, could increase my ability to get around. Thus my feet became my early warning defense system...." By allowing her feet to lead her, she was able to relax and complete the journey safely. She was using her kinesthetic sense.

A third benefit of exercise is its ability to open up a new way of taking in information. Researchers found that most people have one dominant mode, or way, of learning anything. The three modes are visual (through the eyes), auditory (through the ears), and kinesthetic (through a felt bodily sensation).Understanding the different styles of learning is very important. If three people are present in any situation, they will take in information differently depending on their dominant style. A visual person describing an outdoor wedding might provide a lot of detail about what the wedding party wore and decorations. A person who was auditory would focus more on the music, sounds of the birds, and the tone of voice the couple used in exchanging vows. A kinesthetically focused person would describe the event in terms of the temperature of the air, breezes, and the sensation of being in the crowd as a participant in the event. Each one was fully present and observant but focused on a different aspect of the situation. Scientists have proven that we can all learn to expand our ways of interacting with the world by paying attention to the sensory input available in each mode. What this means is that even when vision becomes weaker, we do not need to lose contact with experience. We may need to shift to other sorts of stimuli and pay more attention to sounds and feelings. Exercise helps us to feel our bodies in space more accurately and with more pleasure. It allows us to open up the kinesthetic sense as a way to learn about and participate in our environment. As your vision improves through the use of the other techniques in this book, you will continue to enjoy the benefits of having developed your kinesthetic sense.

The fourth reason to exercise is the same for fully sighted and low vision persons. This is the cardiovascular benefit from aerobic exercise. Simply stated, aerobic exercise makes you breathe harder. Faster breathing speeds up your metabolism and allows you body to rid itself of wastes and toxins. Any form of sustained, fast-paced movement accelerates the heart beat while training it to perform under stress so that it does not beat too fast. In the beginning of an aerobic program, the heart rate is apt to be very fast with only moderate exertion. After a while, the heart rate goes up only slightly with exertion. Monitoring your heart rate while exercising strenuously will give you an idea of how much benefit you are deriving from your exercise program. If you do not have a regular exercise program, now is the time to start.

Exercise

Begin slowly under your physician's supervision by exercising ten to fifteen minutes several times per week. This should gradually be increased to thirty minutes of exercise every day. The ideal exercise program will increase your heart rate moderately without producing fatigue. A general guideline is to exercise at 60% of your maximum heart rate. This is measured during the most intense period of your exercise program. To calculate this number, subtract your age from 220. This number is your maximum heart rate. Sixty percent of this number will be your target heart rate. Aim to exercise in the range between your target rate and your maximum rate. If your heart beats faster than this, there is greater risk of injury to muscles and the heart itself. A good rule of thumb is that when you have difficulty carrying on a conversation, you have reached your target rate.

Heart Rates for Selected Ages

Age	Max Heart Rate	Target Rate
40	180	108
45	175	105
50	170	102
55	165	99
60	160	96
65	155	93
70	150	90

To calculate your target heart rate, exercise to the point where you feel you are putting out a good effort. Stop and take your pulse for 15 seconds. You can feel it easily by placing two fingers on the artery on the side of your neck. Multiply this number by four to obtain your heart rate. If this number is greater than your maximum heart rate, you need to decrease your effort until you reach a state just under your maximum heart rate. This is the most efficient level. It enables you to have to a good aerobic workout the risk of injury. After doing this for a time, you will learn how to recognize when you have achieved your maximum heart rate without checking your pulse. Remember: more is not better; you need to gradually increase your aerobic capacity. Your heart rate is your guide.

What is Aerobic?

Aerobic exercise means a sustained activity that challenges your heart and lungs. There are many types of aerobic exercise, and these can be done at a pace that matches your abilities. Running is a favorite but may not be possible if your vision makes you feel unsteady or your knees or joints are painful. Cycling is a good choice and can be done in a gym or at home on a stationary bike if your vision does not permit outdoor cycling.

Aerobic dance classes can be fun if you find a class where the routines are not varied too frequently and your visual acuity allows you to see the instructor well. Some types of yoga, as we will discuss later, are aerobic. Even house cleaning or washing the car can be a mini-workout.

Older persons need to exercise in order to combat the decline in flexibility and strength that occurs with age. Many injuries can be prevented if a person is agile and strong. The fractures of osteoporosis (bone thinning) are less likely to occur in individuals who have done weight bearing exercise—this means walking or running

Exercise

or doing something that causes the long bones to carry your weight. Strength building with weights can also combat this condition. Ultimately, your self sufficiency requires that you be able to manage tasks required in daily routines. This can be even more critical to independence than the ability to drive.

Types of exercise

There are three main types of exercise. Some types build strength; others focus on endurance; some types emphasize flexibility. Any of these can be considered aerobic. An example of strength-building exercise is weight lifting. This type of exercise usually targets cerain muscles or muscle groups for development. Strength-building exercise should not be done on consecutive days; a day of rest between workouts is necessary to allow for muscles to heal from the workout. Running, cycling, and fast walking, along with cross-country skiing, are examples of endurance-building exercises. Flexibility is the goal in most types of dance and yoga, although they also promote endurance and strength. Ideally, an exercise program should include all three types with an aerobic workout three times per week alternating with a program for flexibility or agility.

Recent findings on the benefit of exercise reveal that less is required to obtain the cardiovascular benefits than was previously thought. A recent study showed that post menopausal women who walked at a moderate rate (three miles per hour) for one hour three times per week had 40 percent less chance of a heart attack than those who did not exercise. You must begin where you are. If you can only walk ten minutes, then do it. Nothing builds faster than the capacity for movement. Even a sedentary person who begins to exercise, will soon start to crave some movement every day. By the way, cleaning out the garage, weeding the garden, and scrubbing floors are all examples of movement. Think of ways to work out while you go about your daily routine. Is it possible to walk to a store or mailbox? Small children will usually get adults outside for walks to the park. Ditto for dogs. Can you borrow a child or a dog to help you work out? The idea in motivating yourself to exercise is to make it enjoyable. If you are person who loves to exercise and focus on it, so much the better. However, many people need to be tricked into exercising while they are doing something else like watching birds or washing the car.

Now that you know how much more a person with low vision person benefits from exercise than a fully sighted person, let's get started! Always consult, not only your ophthalmologist, but your general physician before beginning an exercise program. Your age and physical condition may require you to take certain precautions in exercising. Please be prudent. With respect to ARMD, those who have wet ARMD and tend to bleed must be certain to consult their ophthalmologist before undertaking any strenuous exercise for fear of it impacting the retina itself.

Where to exercise

Finding your place with exercise is key to maintaining a disciplined schedule. The first choice to make is outdoors vs. indoors. Some people rebel against the confinement of a gym or class or even of their own home. If you choose to exercise out of doors, you can design a very adequate program that promotes aerobic fitness and increases your flexibility. It is more difficult to build

Exercise

strength with a program that is exclusively done outdoors. You may want to combine outdoor workouts in fair weather with indoor workouts in foul. Good all-around outdoor activities include fast walking, running, cycling, and cross country skiing. If you are up to skating, both ice and in-line skating are excellent aerobic workouts. Swimming is one of the best conditioning undertakings and can make persons with low vision, feel quite relaxed since vision is not critical to successful swimming.

If you like indoor exercising or need to limit yourself to indoor workouts, the next choice to make is whether to purchase home equipment or go to a gym or both. Working out in a gym has many benefits in general. There is a wider variety of equipment than any home gym could acquire. There are trained staff people to help. It may be possible to take classes in special forms of exercise along with designing your own workout. Aerobic workouts, strength training, and flexibility-building classes can usually be found in one spot.

Persons with limited sight may have special considerations in using a gym, however. Getting to and from the gym and navigating it are things to consider. However, all exercise progresses better when done with a friend or companion. If you find a companion with whom to exercise, consider yourself fortunate. If this person can also help with transportation, assuming you need this help, so much the better.

Working out at home offers the advantage of a familiar surrounding and the possibility of your partner or family member participating. It is limited by the types of workouts you can do. One advantage, though, is that you can purchase videos to instruct you in unfamiliar routines or types of exercise. Usually libraries and video stores have these available for loan, giving you an opportunity to find one you really like before purchasing it.

However, don't expect to be satisfied with one video for too long. If you are making progress, you will want to upgrade from time to time. If your vision is low, a family member can help you assume the positions or do the steps shown on the video while you freeze the action.

Speaking of getting help, consider hiring a coach or personal trainer. A trainer can help you design your program whether you are at home or using a gym. They are accustomed to working with persons at all skill and fitness levels, so don't think you need to be Adonis to use one. They will tailor their work to help you meet your own personal goals. They do not merely show up with a workout for you. By the way, you don't need goals like adding two inches to your biceps. Simply wanting to exercise three times a week and strengthen a sore lower back are good enough to begin.

The Trampoline

Jumping on a trampoline, called "rebounding" has been shown to be one of the most effective and accessible forms of aerobic exercise. All it requires is the purchase of a small exercise trampoline, available in most sporting goods stores. Those who feel unstable can buy a stabilizer bar that attaches to the trampoline, making it easy to use for almost anyone. There are portable models for those who travel or want to take it to work on a daily basis.

The best way to use it is for a total of 30 to 40 minutes per day. These can be in divided sessions or all at one time. Naturally, a beginner will work up to this amount of time over a period of weeks. The technique involves simple jumping. The construction of the trampoline virtually eliminates the possibility of injury to tis-

Exercise

sues, joints, or limbs. It is easy to use inside the house or out of doors. You can watch TV, chat on the phone, or visit with the family while you rebound

Rebounding tones your body, reduces fat, increases energy, and, most importantly, stimulates the immune system. The immune system is composed of lymph nodes and lymph channels. Lymph nodes, located throughout the body, but primarily in the groin and upper chest, store toxins until they can be released through the venous system. Toxins reach the lymph nodes through the action of white blood cells and other specialized cells that attack poisons and foreign material in the body. Unlike the blood, which is pumped by the heart, lymph relies on movement and exercise to circulate. That means that stagnation occurs when you exercise too little. However, rebounding has been found to be extremely efficient in moving lymph. Along with this come the added benefits of a toned immune system.

The aerobic quality of the jumping will raise your heartbeat to your target zone quite quickly without your feeling overly tired or stressed. This will allow you to keep rebounding for a longer time than you could sustain another activity such as jogging. It is gentle, effective, easy to do, and quite inexpensive. What are you waiting for?

Music

We talked about the opportunities involved in opening up your other two ways of taking in the world when vision is low. It can be very pleasurable to combine music with movement. This, of course, is done in dancing, and you may find that dance classes or lessons are a good way to begin getting some exercise. But music can be combined with all forms of working out. Fast music goes with aerobics; slow music can accompany yoga postures. Anything from Hawaiian to classical music can be the background to a free-form dance and movement session of your own design. This is one of the richest ways to enjoy your body and movement.

Yoga

Yoga means union in Sanskrit, union of mind and body. There are many forms of yoga, with some being pure meditation or contemplation. The type of yoga most popular with westerners is hatha yoga. Hatha yoga classes offer an hour or more of rather slow movement while you assume various postures as instructed by the yoga teacher. These postures are held while lying down, sitting, and standing up. Yoga is usually practiced in one place on a mat, so there is no need to navigate unfamiliar territory. A bonus to visually impaired people is that it is usually done with closed eyes. Yoga really helps you to feel your body and can be a wonderful alternative to more vigorous forms of exercise. It is unparalleled in producing flexibility. Every yoga class allows some time for complete relaxation which, as we will see in the next chapter, is one of the most important components of good health. Another benefit of yoga is its emphasis on correct and rhythmic breathing. A very good class in yoga is apt to be offered at your local senior center or adult education program. There are videos available to help you use this technique at home also.

There are several types of yoga. This brief review may be helpful to you in choosing a form that is best. Iyengar yoga is a type of hatha yoga that emphasizes strength as well as flexibility. The postures have a very definite form and are maintained longer than those in simple hatha yoga. Kundalini yoga is highly aerobic with deep and sometimes fast breathing. It can be quite a workout, but it still incorporates relaxation. Bikram yoga uses the same series of postures in a fluid, aerobic workout from class to class. Classes are held in superheated rooms to promote flexibility.

Water Workouts

As we mentioned earlier, water is a good medium for visually impaired persons since it does not require good sight. Many YMCA's have programs of aquathenics or water ballet for people with stressed joints, injuries, or arthritis. Water is a very forgiving medium for movement since form is not so important and one does not feel fatigued after a session. Swimming, of course, can also be a rewarding sport, and, along with ice skating, is unparalleled in working many muscle groups without needing to focus on any one in particular.

Oriental Forms Of Exercise

In both China and Japan, it is common to see groups of people, whether employees, students, or residents of the same apartment building, performing rhythmic movements each morning. Quite likely the real purpose of these movements can only be revealed by studying the ancient teachings of the cultures. One cannot help but notice that this seems like a peaceful way to greet the day. (Compare it to grabbing a coffee and doughnut on the way into an American office building.) It also seems to speak to a certain solidarity or unity among the people exercising together. Since it is usually done out of doors in the morning, it seems to relate people to nature at the beginning of a new day.

Several forms of exercise that originated in the orient are becoming very popular in the United States. Tai Chi is perhaps the best known. It requires participants to assume various postures very slowly and deliberately in an effort to enhance balance and grace. It is thought that the inner currents of energy are freed to move in a more healing and unobstructed way as a result of this practice. QiGong is another form of movement especially favored by the elderly in China. These techniques can be found on videos, if you have no classes in your area. Done slowly and with the use of appropriate support, such as chair back to hold onto for balance, they are safe and rewarding. Senior centers may offer these classes, and there they will be paced to those who need assistance and must move a bit more slowly. Like yoga, these practices also focus on the peaceful interplay of mind and body.

Synergy

This book offers twelve steps to help you improve your ARMD. Actually, that is not a large number of things to do. It may, at first, seem overwhelming. Think of ways to combine some of these suggestions. For example, growing some of your own food will ensure its high quality while providing an opportunity for exercise in the garden. In the next chapter, we are going to talk about relaxation. Several of the exercise methods we mentioned here, namely yoga and Tai Chi, focus on having a relaxed mind. However, all forms of exercise have been shown to reduce anxiety and depression. If you have become

Exercise

dependent on cigarettes or caffeine, which we will talk about in a later chapter, you need to give them up. Exercise as well as stress reduction will help you kick these bad habits. A good diet will lessen your craving for unhealthy substances. So, think synergy. Select those activities that help you redesign your life in ways that make sense for your situation and have the greatest payoff in terms of rebuilding your health.

Four Reasons to Exercise

♦ Fight Depression

    ♦ Improve confidence; increase safety

♦ Develop kinesthetic sense

    ♦ Improve cardiovascular health

Check List for Step Three

√ Select a type of exercise that appeals to you.

√ Find a place to exercise.

√ Find an exercise partner.

√ Learn to monitor your heart rate.

√ Begin to exercise three times per week.

√ Introduce variety into your routine.

Exercise

Step 4

Cope With Stress

I am going to begin this chapter with a very short quiz—one question in fact. Do you have stress in your life? You do not need to turn the page upside down to find the answer. There is only one correct answer and that is "no." Are you surprised? Perhaps, like many of my patients, you want to say, "Dr. Kondrot, you just don't know about my life. It is full of stress, and there isn't a thing I can do about it. There's the job or the lack of a job, the teenagers, the in-laws, my aging parents, traffic...." Yes, I've heard all about it. But here is the secret: there is no such thing as stress; there is only life. Stress comes into the picture in the way we respond to events.

You've probably heard something to the effect that the only real freedom we have is in how to respond to whatever life presents. We cannot control it. In fact, trying to control events or people produces inner tension and anxiety. The only thing we can control is our response. Think about it. Even in a very frightful situation, for example if your neighbor's house is consumed by flames, you can still choose how to respond. You can pitch in and help douse the flames. You can take in the poor neighbors and offer tea and comfort. You can loan your neighbors your phone and car to cope with their immediate needs. You can just keep reading the newspaper or watching TV. You can stand in the street and wring your hands with your heart and mind racing. What is the most appropriate response? From a social standpoint, any helpful response is appropriate. And most of us would be able to understand the hand-wringing. From a health standpoint, any response that keeps your vital signs steady is a good one. Therefore, continuing to watch TV is okay. (Studies have shown, however, that social involvement is a real plus in longevity, so ignoring your neighbors might not actually be healthy in the overall sense.) The impulse to fight the flames stems from a desire to contain the fire but also from your body's need to stabilize your vital signs. Accelerated heart rate and respiration are two of the physiological responses to tense situations, and activity is a way to normalize them. This is the flight or fight response you have probably learned about. Less talked about but equally important is the freeze response. This is also a natural reaction (think about rabbits!) to danger, and some people will freeze while others flee or fight.

You Can Choose Your Response

As you can see, we can choose our response regardless of the situation. Driving provides an interesting example because all drivers in one area are dealing with the same set of conditions. One driver will pull out of the driveway with a squeal of tires, and a blast of rock music, all set for road rage at the slightest obstacle. The next will nose out slowly, knuckles whitened on the wheel, squinting because vision is low, creeping along below the speed limit, and exhausted after just a few minutes of coping with the many choices driving requires. Each driver is exhibiting a stress response. The first one is related to fight or flight, and the second is freezing. A third driver will drive in an aware but highly relaxed state. She will signal to other drivers to proceed whenever there is an opportunity. She smiles at them too. She is aware of traffic flow in determining her speed and is just naturally alert to special circumstances that require evasive or assertive driving. Remember that all three of these drivers are apt to be in the same group of cars at one stoplight. In other words, they are all dealing with the same external conditions, but their internal response to these conditions shapes the way they react.

Let's examine this a little further. Driver number one may have a number of physiological contributors to his driving style. Caffeine is a suspect, perhaps even amphetamines or some other stimulating drug. Maybe he just finished an argument with a house mate or partner that left his adrenaline pumping before jumping into the car. Thoughts about an early morning meeting with his boss keep him on edge because he has been late turning in his reports recently. Speaking of being late, he left the house with no time to spare to get to work. However, if we look a little deeper into his life, we see that all these situations have developed because of the same pattern— the tendency to live on the edge, cut corners, and focus on himself to the exclusion of others' needs.

Driver number two also has contributing factors to her tendency to freeze. She takes a few prescription drugs that slow down her reflexes, so she is always somewhat depressed. Lately, she has been getting lost, even in familiar neighborhoods, so she is concentrating very intensely on her driving that is difficult because she cannot see all that well. Although her daughter-in-law offered to take her to her appointment today, she refused help because she wants to prove to herself and everyone else that she is still independent, not failing in any way. We might notice how driver number two also focuses on her needs to the exclusion of others. She is not a safe driver, but she insists on driving to prove a point. While we may feel more sympathy for the second driver, she is, in some ways, as antisocial as the first driver.

Balance is the Goal

The third driver exhibits balance. She can focus well on driving and perform the necessary maneuvers, but she is not consumed by the task. Nor is she distracted by other aspects of her life. It appears that events that occurred before she left home as well as the situation she is likely to find at her destination cause her little concern. She is the picture of balance and peace. This is not to say that everything in her life is balanced and peaceful. Far from it. In fact, she is very worried that her younger brother might be into drugs. She knows he has an appointment with his boss today and is in danger of losing his job. Silently she offers a brief prayer that he will be given another chance if that is in his best interest. If his getting fired is the wake-up call he needs, she hopes that he will learn from it. She is also aware that her mother-in-law has a doctor appointment today. When she notices herself feeling tense because the older woman rejected her offer of help, she lets go of that thought. Instead she reaffirms that she cannot control another's behavior. After that, she sends an inner message of peace to her mother-in-law and hopes that the day goes well for her. While she is about it, she sends love and peace to her husband who was angry with her this morning because she had not insisted on accompanying his mother to the doctor. She makes a mental note to give him a back rub after dinner. Just then she pulls into the parking lot of her company and prepares for a meeting with the auditor who informed her that one of her employees may be embezzling. "Well," she thinks, "this is a challenge I've never had to face before. I'm sure to learn a lot."

Creating Emotional Distance

If we examine the reactions of the three people described above, we might say that the first two are very close, in an emotional sense, to their situations while the third person has the ability to allow some space between her and her life. This space can be mental or emotional or even physical. For example, she allows herself to feel that there is hope for her brother whether or not he

Cope with Stress

loses his job. She distances herself from the situation enough that either outcome can be seen as a good one. Her brother, on the other hand, feels that his life will be ruined if he is fired. She also acknowledges her mother-in-law's right to refuse help. Although our third driver does not actually think her mother-in-law can cope well with the doctor visit, she realizes that she cannot force herself on the older woman. She is aware that her husband is investigating ways to assume more stewardship for his mother through legal processes, but, until this is in place, the older woman is free to make her own decisions. She can also anticipate that the situations of both her brother and mother-in-law are apt to evoke some very unpleasant feelings in all the family members, including herself. By rehearsing and preparing for her own reactions, she hopes to be calmer when the new developments emerge. These types of thoughts give her perspective, one of the ways she gives herself space and more freedom to choose her responses.

How did this woman learn to stay relaxed despite events in her life? Chances are she did it for the same reasons you are interested in doing it. She reached a point where her stressful reactions to life began to cause her physical problems. Perhaps she suffered from migraine headaches, insomnia, or high blood pressure. Some people exhibit mental and emotional symptoms from stress. Perhaps she used to be irritable, anxious, or depressed a significant amount of the time. Her ability to enjoy life became tainted with worry and anxiety regarding the future, and she decided to do something about it.

Regardless of what prompted her to change, we might observe that she has succeeded in mastering herself.

What is Stress?

Stress is the body's reaction to stressors, those provoking events that cause us to become disturbed and feel off balance. Once we differentiate between stressors and stress, we can learn to say, "I have many stressors but not much stress." If stressors are outside of us, where is stress? Stress is actually the term for our physiological response to events in our environment. These events can affect us in the physical, mental, or emotional level. For example, a long-lasting cold or bout with the flu stresses us physically. An argument stresses us emotionally. Worry and anxiety stress us mentally. Stress is very simply our autonomic (means the same as automatic) nervous system's response to events. We have two nervous systems. One is the set of nerves and impulses that control our voluntary functions like posture and movement. This is under our voluntary control. For example, when we decide to move a leg, we do it. We may not spend much time thinking about it, but we know that we can make ourselves move as well as stop ourselves from moving.

However, a large number of our bodily processes are not under our voluntary control. These include digestion, the secretion of hormones from our glands, and the blood flow though our blood vessels to name a few. These are the very processes most affected by stressors. A stress reaction is nothing but our organism perceiving

Cope with Stress

and reacting to danger.

In primitive life, humans needed to use the extra energy created from stress responses to defend themselves. The ability to flee from wild animals or fires, to pursue and kill dangerous prey were life-preserving activities of our forebears. Today, very few of us encounter life or death challenges on a daily basis. However, because our minds exaggerate the danger of ordinary events, our bodies continue to respond in their primitive life-preserving way. Although it is possible to be maimed or even killed by another automobile, cars are not actually out to get us.. If a driver believes every car in his range of vision is potentially lethal, he will drive in a state of hyper-alertness and with aggression that keeps his primitive life-preserving juices flowing full force. Any number of everyday events can trigger the autonomic nervous system to turn on full blast. Situations at work, job interviews, encounters with our teenagers, or visits to the doctor or dentist cause many people so much worry and anxiety that they shift into high gear emotionally and physiologically. Following is a list of bodily reactions that occur during stress, taken from Kenneth Pelletier's fine work on the subject, *Mind as Healer, Mind as Slayer.*

> Give me the *courage* to change what can be changed,
> the *serenity* to accept what cannot be changed,
> and the *wisdom* to know the difference

Physical Components of the Stress Response

Dilated pupils
Tight throat
Tense neck and upper back
Shallow respiraion
Accelerated heart rate
Cool, perspiring hands
A locked diaphragm
A rigid pelvis with numb genitals

All of these reactions serve to preserve our body when it is under attack. What is going on internally is that blood flow to the extremities and the gastro-intestinal area is reduced and more blood is sent to the head and trunk in order to preserve the most important organs. This is a very good adaptation the human body has developed in order to survive life threatening situations. The problem is that the pace and intensity of modern life have caused us to call on this capacity many, many times a day. In fact, research has shown that simply thinking of a tense or highly unpleasant situation causes the very same response in the body. Many times we experience this state without even knowing why we feel anxious. So-called subliminal stimuli (those we do not focus on) can produce the stress reaction. Examples of subliminal stimuli are violent or gory images, constant background noise, and noxious odors.

Cope with Stress

How Stress makes You Sick

The bodily changes I described above, while necessary to preserve life in an emergency, are very harmful to the body when they occur frequently or are maintained for long periods of time. This last point is worth exploring. When our primitive forebears experienced the flight, fight, or freeze response, they did not need to stay in that situation for long. Either they killed the wild animal or it killed them. However, in modern life it is not uncommon for people to live in a mildly stressed state virtually every waking minute. It is unlikely that their sleep will be restful after a day on hyper-alert either. So, even at night, the processes of repair and recuperation are compromised by a stress reaction that never lets up. Is it any surprise that feeling tired is our most frequent complaint as a society? We have even developed the disease named Chronic Fatigue Syndrome.

If you look at the list of physical stress reactions listed above, you can easily translate them into difficulties that plague. Complaints like neck and back pain, tense shoulders, digestive problems, menstrual disorders and sexual difficulties, cold hands and feet are all symptomatic of the autonomic nervous system's excessive involvement. Hypertension, migraine headache, irritable bowel syndrome are all examples of the body taking on a chronic stressed response. Many people have multiple complaints of this sort.

Stress and Eye Disease

Stress is related to many eye complaints. In his book, *The Cure of Imperfect Sight by Treatment Without Glasses,* Dr. William Bates states that the cause of all problems is stress. Stress produces tightness in the muscles of the eye. This tightness in some way blocks the energy flow to the eye and may result in disease. You may notice that under stress, your eye begins to ache or you may have trouble focusing. These symptoms are the early signs of eye stress. If this is not dealt with properly, it can lead to eye disease such as cataract, glaucoma, ARMD, or even a stroke involving the eye. Throughout my years of practice, I have observed patients develop serious eye problems after stress-producing events. The death of a loved one, the loss of a job, retirement, and other events may affect someone so much that the body 'does not want to see' what has happened. This response is then focused in the eye and a visual problem will develop. I have noticed that the death of a loved one may lead to cataract development. Even the sudden change of retiring or losing a job can result in ARMD. We all respond to stress differently, and, unfortunately, the eye is often the point of the body where the steam from the pressure cooker is released.

The Relaxation Response

Over thirty years ago, Hans Selye wrote the first widely-read book about stress called *Stress Without Dis-*

tress. He was a researcher at Harvard who performed some of first tests that measured stress in the body. He also suggested that if we could engage our stress response, perhaps we could engage something he called the "Relaxation Response." This refers to a deliberate and conscious attempt to delay or slow down the stress response and bring it under voluntary control. The concept involved three steps: learning how to relax the body deliberately, doing it on a regular basis, and bringing this learned response into play whenever stressors are encountered.

Much of Dr. Selye's work focused on some of the ancient systems of bodily control exhibited by the yogis of the east who were famous for walking on beds of nails and swallowing fire. It turned out that they could do these things because they had control over bodily responses and processes thought to be beyond voluntary control. The perception of pain is an example. While Selye and others who studied this subject were not interested in helping people develop extraordinary powers of yogis, they wanted to help people gain more control of their bodies.

It turned out that the breath is the link between the part of our nervous system we can control and the part we cannot control. Think about it. You can control your breath if you choose. However, if you don't think about it, or even if you are unconscious, you keep breathing. Since hyperventilation is also a stress reaction, it was suggested that if that process could be brought under control through slow deep breathing, the rest of the autonomic nervous system would disengage the stress response. Therefore, the breath is considered to be a key to the relaxation response. Most of us know that the reminder to take a breath or breathe slowly in a tense situation can actually calm us.

A second key to relaxation is visualization. Biofeedback is a technique used to help people control things like intractable pain, migraine headaches, and hypertension by training them to focus on the area involved and relax it. During Biofeedback sessions, patients are monitored by electronic equipment and their responses are measured. This allows them to observe their effectiveness in controlling their bodily processes. For example, people with migraine headaches caused by constricted blood vessels can find relief if they focus on their hands getting warmer. The theory is that they are actually dilating their blood vessels throughout their body. Some people do this by visualizing and others through their kinesthetic sense. Just as I mentioned that thinking about a stressful event can cause a stress reaction, just imagining a relaxed state can produce it. You do not need to study texts on the body/mind connection to prove this to yourself.

We owe a great deal to the early research done in the area of relaxation. In fact, all the newer work has been built on this concept. The challenge now is not to prove that we need to learn to relax voluntarily or to demonstrate that we can learn how to do it. The challenge is to convince people that this is not only worthwhile, but necessary for their well being. We cannot control the world. Natural disasters, horrible crimes, accidents, and personal losses will still occur with regularity. I strongly recommend that you review the following ways to learn how to relax and incorporate one into your life without delay.

Six Ways to Relax

1. Abdominal breathing

This technique is so simple and effective that it will become addictive. You will find yourself seeking a quiet corner wherever you are to practice it. You do not need to purchase anything either! Twice a day, for 15-20 minutes, lie down on the floor, sofa, or bed and breathe deeply while staying awake. Stretch out in a comfortable position on your back, bending your knees and putting your feet on the floor. Place your hands on your lower belly, below the navel. Breathe slowly into your abdomen so that your hands move up and down gently. Stay awake but very relaxed. You may, if you wish, do progressive relaxation. This entails relaxing each part of the body in turn from the head down. This can help you stay awake. Of course, you do not need to feel like a failure if you do doze off. Consider yourself a master of the power nap!

2. Affirmations

This method of relaxing is completely different from the one above. They can be combined easily, however. Our minds are responsible for a lot of our stressed reaction to life. We worry and obcess about the future and about things we cannot control in any way. We also give ourselves negative messages about our capabilities and appearance on a regular basis. A diet of this erodes self-esteem. A lack of self esteem can convince us that we cannot cope with events. You see how this produces a never-ending cycle.

Replace your negative thoughts with a positive thought. If you try to do this every time you have a negative thought, you will probably get into arguing with yourself. For example, if you were planning to attend a class reunion, your mind might say, "They are all going to notice how much you've aged." Then your mind must say something like, "I've lived my life as well as I could, and if I look older, so be it." Then another part of your mind will say, "But you could have lost a few pounds for the reunion." See how it goes? You get nowhere. The way to replace your negative thoughts is to come up with a universal, comprehensive, positive statement that is true for you. Once you have this worked out, say it to yourself all the time. That's right: say it all the time. Say it in the shower, driving the car, vacuuming; say it whenever your mind is not concentrating on something worthwhile. Believe me, this is a lot of the time. Once you begin to do this, you will also notice how useless and repetitious most of your thoughts are.

You may have heard the statement that the late Dale Carnegie is said to have repeated to himself daily. "Every day in every way, I am getting better and better." We tend to laugh at this because it sounds a little egotistical. But think about it. How often do we tell ourselves just the reverse in constant, nagging inner chatter full of doubts and negativity.

Cope with Stress

Some people are able to feel comfortable saying something like, "I always do my best." This does not mean you are perfect; it simply states the truth that you do the best you can. Statements like, "My heart is full of love for all" create a wonderful mental atmosphere. If you are spiritually oriented or religious, you can say something like, "I am always guided and protected." Remember: keep it simple; keep it positive. Do not say something like, "I will not think negative thoughts." Rather, say, "My mind now focuses on the positive." See the difference? Also, make your affirmation believable. If saying "I respond with love to all around me" causes a small "Oh, yeah?" response in your mind, then step it down to something you can believe. Perhaps, "I bring more love into my encounters" feels more appropriate.

The important thing is to choose an affirmation and get started with it. Say it all the time. Write it on post-it notes and post them around the house. After a while, you will want to change it. Feel free; it is your affirmation. What will this technique do for you? First, it takes up mental space so that your negative thoughts have no room. Secondly, it fills the mental space with peaceful and powerful messages that keep the autonomic nervous system relaxed because it does not sense any danger.

3. Meditate

Meditation is a technique to quiet the mind and relax the body on a regular basis. For some people, it has spiritual overtones because if you are not experiencing yourself as a mind or a body, who are you? People who meditate come into contact with the timeless and formless sense of themselves. This is truly relaxing and highly desirable for many reasons. Although there are many types of meditation, all types focus on relaxation through awareness of the breath and emptying the mind of thoughts. Many people find this very difficult to do. I will try to give you some tips that may relieve the pressure if you are just learning to meditate. Of course, there are many wonderful meditation teachers who can work with you individually, and I suggest you find one if you are drawn to do so. It is also true that a form of meditation is usually included in yoga classes because it is easier to meditate when you are physically relaxed. If you learn to do this in yoga classes, you can practice the same techniques at home.

4. Relax your body

People new to meditation are usually daunted by the advice to "sit in a relaxed posture on the floor with your spine completely straight and your legs crossed." Most of us do not spend much time sitting this way in our daily life, and it feels uncomfortable. It is just fine to sit in a chair, with a pillow supporting your back, and your feet flat on the floor. Or sit on the sofa and cross your legs. The goal is to stay erect and comfortable without going to sleep.

Cope with Stress

5. Relax your mind.

Worse than the fight with the body is the fight with the mind! Thoughts seem to cascade through your consciousness just when you want none at all. This is another good time for your affirmation. You see, sophisticated as it is, your mind can only hold one thought at a time. If you are thinking "I am now relaxed," thoughts about whether it is time to change the oil in your car cannot intrude! With practice, you will find little islands of time appear when you are not saying your affirmation and you are not thinking about anything else. That's great. Consider it natural when your mind suddenly realizes it has switched off and kicks into high gear like a drowning person taking a first breath. Just go back to the affirmation. Be gentle with yourself.

6. Control your breath.

We have already demonstrated the importance of controlling the breath as a way to control the stress response. Controlling the breath is also an integral part of meditation. Just as you may experience moments without thought, you may find that you require fewer breaths while meditating. You will be able to go for several seconds without breathing. This is fine and normal when it happens, but do not force it. Focusing on the breath is a way to control the mind. Since it can handle only one thought at a time, if it is thinking about breathing, it won't think about anything else.

Evoking Relaxation instead of Stress

All of the techniques I have described can be considered training. You are training your body and mind to be relaxed and, ultimately, to relax on command. It is virtually impossible to relax on command when events provoke you, and you have no practice with relaxation. However, with daily practice in controlling your mind and calming your body, you will find that you have a much less intense reaction to whatever your life presents. You will begin to experience the space our third driver was able to put between herself and her problems: peace.

In the next chapter we will explore methods to relax your eyes specifically. The more practice you have in total body relaxation, the more proficient you will become in the eye exercises. Keep up the good work.

Checklist for Step Four

√   Identify your typical stress Response:
Fight, Flight, or Freeze

√   Identify a daily stress trigger in your life

√   Choose a relaxation method

√   Relax consciously twice daily

√   Memorize the six ways to relax

- Abdominal Breathing
- Affirmation
- Meditation
- Relax the Body
- Relax the Mind
- Breathe Consciously

Step 5 | Exercise and Relax Your Eyes

In the two previous chapters, we have talked about building a daily routine of general exercise and relaxation. Now I want you to enhance that by including a special routine for your eyes. You need not do your eye exercises and relaxation at the same time as your other workouts. In fact, you will find it really easy to build the eye routines into many other parts of your day, such as driving or riding in a car, any type of waiting experience, or sitting in almost any room of your home at any time in the day. It's that easy! The important thing is to make a commitment to this and do it. I know you will want to do so after reading the rest of this chapter.

How Eye Doctors Can Harm You

No doubt you are familiar with having your eyesight tested. You enter a darkened room with the examiner who uses a very large piece of equipment to gaze at the inner parts of your eye through the pupil (the black part in the center). To make the examination go more smoothly, the doctor puts drops in your eyes to make the pupil expand, or dilate. This usually makes it very difficult to focus on anything with clarity. Prior to putting the drops in your eyes, you are usually asked to read an eye chart on the wall with several lines of letters where each lower line gets smaller. Depending on how many lines you can read, the doctor knows how to express your vision in terms of a fraction. If your vision is 20/20, it is considered perfect. What this actually means is that at a distance of 20 feet, you can see what the test subjects could see at 20 feet. If your vision is 20/40, this means that at 20 feet, you can see what these people saw at 40 feet. If it is 20/100, they could see at 100 feet, what you can see at 20 feet. A score of 20/200 and greater, means you are legally blind. After the measurement is taken, you will be given a prescription for 'corrective' lenses, either glasses or contact lenses to wear in order to bring your vision as close as possible to 20/20.

This way of taking care of our eyes is rarely challenged or even questioned. The whole profession of eye care experts, including ophthalmologists and optometrists seems to be so well intentioned and so progressive, not to mention effective, that for the most part we follow their recommendations blindly you might say. And they are indeed well-meaning individuals. The question I began to ask myself and that I would like you to ask yourself is about effectiveness. For example, corrective lenses really don't correct anything. They help you compensate for defective eyesight, but do nothing to help you recover from it or strengthen your eyes. In fact, most people who use glasses find that they must get ever-stronger prescriptions to help them see. In other words, perhaps the idea that you can reverse problems in vision is a new one to you. It is not, however, a new one in history.

William Bates was born in Newark, New Jersey, in 1860. He was a well trained ophthalmologist of the day who, in addition to his practice, lectured and wrote articles. It is in his book, *Perfect Sight Without Glasses,* that he explains his simple but revolutionary theory of vision. The foundation of his theory revolved around these four statements, as summarized by Peter Mansfield in his excellent book, *The Bates Method*:

- Normal sight is inherently variable.
- Defective sight can get better as well as worse.
- Poor sight and eye disease are intimately related.
- Eyesight is an important indicator of mental, emotional, and physical health.

I'd like to discuss these tenets one at a time. The first one—the idea that normal sight is inherently variable—points to one of the greatest flaws in our testing protocol. We eye doctors literally 'freeze' a person in time and space and take a measurement of something that, by its nature, is fluid and ever changing. Dr. Bates demonstrated, using an earlier version of the very same ophthalmoscope we use today, that the eye makes continual minuscule accommodations in order to see. This explains why people are so often dissatisfied with their eyeglasses. They are intended to 'correct' the eyesight so that the person wearing them can see an eye chart in a darkened room. Very few life situations simulate the exam room conditions. Many people find their glasses too strong to wear in bright light, for example. Some people feel dizzy when they wear glasses. This is because the glasses work best when we stare straight ahead at a stationary object and keep absolutely still.

The second radical statement Bates made is that defective sight can get better as well as worse. This means that persons who are near-sighted (myopic) and far-sighted (hyperopic) as well as those with other conditions can improve their vision. They may come to a point where they do not need their glasses or that they need them only under certain conditions. The distinction is between something that is a mechanical aid vs. something that is part of their anatomy! One of the ways this happens is through strengthening the muscles involved in sight and the other is in re-training the eyes to see more effectively.

If you have ARMD, you know that poor sight and disease are intimately related. But, if you are among the many people who had myopia for many years before developing ARMD, I bet you never thought of your nearsightedness as a disease. Yet we now know that myopia, hyperopia, presbyopia, astigmatism, lazy eye, and crossed eyes are all conditions that reveal fundamental weakness in the affected eyes. We also know that these conditions can be reversed to a great extent through vision training and the other techniques Bates recommended.

Looking at the last tenet, that eyesight and overall health are intimately related, gives us hope. Healing the eye heals the whole person. That's why I can say with assurance that following the twelve steps suggested in this book will provide you with the highest level of health you have ever had!

The Difference Between Eyesight and Vision

I strongly suggest that you read one of the books mentioned in the resources section for this chapter in order to more fully grasp the revolutionary ideas of Dr. Bates. Fortunately he translated his complex theories into practical exercises that are very easy to do and that will work whether or not you know the theories behind them. However, there is just one theory that seems very important to explain before I give you the exercises for vision training. This is the idea that eyesight and vision are entirely different. Eyesight is the measurement that results from the testing procedure described above. No doubt you are familiar with this and most likely know what your eyesight measures in each eye. Now, if we took two people with the same eyesight and put them through a series of tests of their *vision*, I am willing to bet that their ability to see would differ significantly. This is because seeing or vision is a result of much more than the mechanics of the eye. It includes memory, experience, and emotions. It is also a function of how relaxed you are at any one time and how accepting you are of what you see. Exploring the role of all these factors is the approach Dr. Bates took and is the basis of the techniques of vision training that are widely available today. I want to emphasize how empowering this understanding of the difference between eyesight and vision can be to you. You may have the experience that many of my patients have had. They do their exercises faithfully and discover that they can see much better. When they come back to me for an exam, I tell them that their eyesight is the same. That means that they are still reading the same line in the chart. However, I fully believe it when they tell me that they can see better, because I now understand that there is a lot more to seeing than meets the eye!

Aldous Huxley Meets Dr. Bates

You may be surprised to learn that one of great philosophers of this century, Aldous Huxley, benefited enormously from the method of eye treatment that I will be describing in this chapter. Mr. Huxley's eye problems were due to an acute infection that left him blind for eighteen months and with the most limited vision after that. Even that began to fail in later years. In desperation he began work with a vision training specialist, a woman who was an associate of Dr. Bates and a founder of the Bates Method. After several months, Mr. Huxley was reading without glasses and had much improved his vision. Problems of twenty-five years' duration were improving. In gratitude for his own experience, he wrote *The Art of Seeing* in 1942 (now out of print, unfortunately) which relates the Bates Method of visual education with modern psychology and critical philosophy. The following quotation from his preface gives an idea of how he saw this work in the context of standard medical practice of his day, over fifty years ago. The following passage is taken from *The Art of Seeing*.

Why, it may be asked, have ophthalmologists failed to make these applications of universally accepted principles? The answer is clear. Ever since ophthalmology became a science, its practitioners have been obsessively preoccupied with only one aspect of the total, complex process of seeing – the physiological. They have paid attention exclusively to eyes, not at all to the mind which makes use of the eyes to see with. I have been treated by men of the highest eminence in their profession, but never once did they so much as faintly hint that there might be a mental side to vision, or that there might be wrong ways of using the eyes and mind as well as right ways, unnatural and abnormal modes of visual functioning as well as natural and normal ones.

———————————

Perhaps your experience has been the same as Huxley's. Up until now, no one has suggested that there might be a better way to use your eyes. Welcome to a new world. I am going to outline a simple vision training program that you can begin doing today, in your own home, without purchasing anything! I know you will find that your ability to see improves.

Exercise and Relax your Eyes

Vision Therapy

In the following sections, I am going to describe some simple and highly enjoyable techniques for stabilizing and improving your vision. These are adapted from the techniques outlined by William Bates. As you approach the task of adopting these as part of your lifestyle, remember that there are three stages. In the first stage, your task will be to learn the techniques. There are a number of ways to help yourself do this. You might record the instructions on a tape recorder as you read through them. Speak slowly, and then play the tape back for yourself as you use the techniques. Since these techniques are good for a variety of eye problems as well as for general eye health, ask a family member or friend to do them with you. Then you can read the instructions to each other, doubling the effect of your effort.

The next state of involvement with the techniques is the initial period of rapid progress. Your poor eyes have been starved, in a sense, for the type of relaxation and stimulation these techniques provide. Naturally, they are apt to respond rapidly during the first few months of workouts. After this, you will probably reach a plateau where you can maintain the gains you achieved, but do not see much more improvement. This is a good time to stabilize your ongoing program and work it into your life on a daily basis. After a time at the plateau stage, you will most likely reach a point where you find yourself making noticeable progress again. Remember, just like exercising and relaxing the body, these techniques are meant to become part of your life forever!

82

The Bates Exercises and ARMD

Traditional Bates exercises form a sound basis for working with retinal damage especially of the kind found in ARMD. The combination of stimulation and relaxation in sunning and palming complement the stimulation and movement found in the practices of swinging and shifting. It very commonly happens that one eye is affected earlier or to a greater extent than the other. Loss of sight in one eye of course can be an even greater cause of strain than the loss of acuity per se, especially if the dominant eye is most affected

The adaptations of Dr Bates' approach which I have developed address the problems of unequal binocular vision. Besides ARMD, these have proved useful in many cases of other conditions such as amblyopia (uniocular and binocular), cataract, strabismus, and all forms of refractive error.

Eye Relaxation And Focusing Exercises

I am indebted for some of the following information to Peter Mansfield, one of Europe's most distinguished Bates Vision Teachers. Peter is Secretary of the Bates Association for Vision Education and Director of the School of Vision Education in England, and teaches privately in Brighton and London. His book, *The Bates Method,* (1992) is published in the USA by Charles Tuttle and in England by Random House. His new book, *Seeing: A Handbook of Vision Education*, is planned for publication in 2000.

83

Exercise and Relax your Eyes

Do all the following exercises without wearing your glasses or sunglasses, in good light. Your glasses or contact lenses prevent your eyes from reaching their capacity by bringing things to them. The purpose of the techniques described below is to enhance your eyes' ability to see. At first you may feel anxious without your glasses, especially if you are in the habit of wearing them all the time. Be sure that you feel safe and secure and are not required to do anything like drive or cook or watch over a young child while you are doing your vision training techniques; this will reduce your anxiety. All three exercises—palming, sunning, and swinging—should be done for 10 to 15 minutes twice a day or more frequently if your doctor advises it.

Palming

The purpose of this technique is to provide total rest for the eyes. Once you have done palming for a while, you will be better able to feel eye strain. All people with impaired sight strain their eyes in their attempt to see better. Palming allows you to develop a relaxed sense so that the other exercises can proceed more smoothly.

Palming is done while sitting at a table with the eyes closed. Rest the elbows on the table and position slightly 'cupped' hands over the eyes, with your fingers crossed on the forehead. The elbows should be supported so that the back is comfortably straight and so that there is no undue pressure on the neck, shoulders and arms. Be aware also of the importance of the position of the feet in achieving a relaxed and comfortable posture.

PALMING

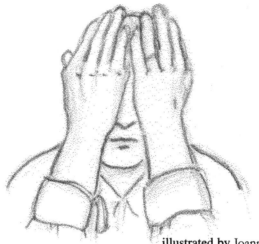

illustrated by Joanne Lew '99

Palming is an excellent way to rest and heal your eyes. You have everything you need with you at all times. I have seen remarkable results in terms of vision improvement in patients who have done this exercise as their only form of treatment. Anyone can practice it, and it is highly recommended as a way of preventing serious eye disease.

Exercise and Relax your Eyes

Do not touch your eyes with your hands. The hands touch only the bony eye sockets. All light is sealed out. In this way, you will begin to recognize the feeling of relaxed eyes. There may be firm contact between hands and face (avoid excessive pressure) but none at all between hands and eyes. Do this exercise at least twice a day, working up to fifteen minutes each time. It is worth experimenting very carefully to find the best position as a very small difference in the height of support can have a big effect on comfort.

Quick Palming

Quick Palming is a variation on the palming technique which is particularly suitable for ARMD patients. It avoids any risk of inadvertently putting sustained pressure on the eyes and combines stimulation with relaxation. Sit relaxed with the eyes closed. Place the hands, palm upwards, in the lap. Feel the flow of energy from the eyes through the face and neck, down the arms and into the upturned hands. Feel the connection between the open palms and the eyes, wanting to complete the circuit. Continue to feel that energetic connection as you slowly raise the hands to the face, sitting upright and using the arms, without hunching the body. Let the hands approach the face very slowly, so that it feels like a sunset as they eventually wrap around bringing warmth and darkness. Hold the hands in position just as long as it is comfortable. Before the arms begin to tire, release the palms from the eyes and again slowly return the hands to the lap. Repeat as often and for as long as you feel that it is helpful.

Swinging

The 'long standing swing' is arguably the most important single practice in the Bates Method. It teaches overall relaxation and helps break the weaker eye's habit of staring fixedly at a point. Swinging produces the illusion that objects are moving. Repeated exposure to this phenomenon of apparent movement will encourage a sense of free mobility and improved vision.

Stand with feet shoulder-width apart. Be sure to wear comfortable supportive shoes. Allow your arms to hang naturally at your side. In one movement, turn your upper body from the waist so that you are facing to one side. This is a 90 degree turn of the body. Keep your head and neck aligned with your shoulders. Eyes are always looking straight ahead. Immediately twist back to starting position, and then to the other direction. As you swing, shift your weight from one foot to the other. The movement should not be greater than ninety degrees from the straight ahead position, and may be less if the full movement causes discomfort.

A slight variation on the simple swing is to use the thumb as a reference point. To do this, follow the directions above, but hold your arm in front of you with your thumb up. Look at your thumb while doing the swing. This will enhance the sensation of apparent movement as your thumb appears to stay still while the background is moving.

SWINGING - RIGHT AND LEFT SIDES

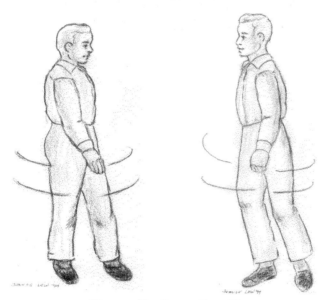

illustrated by Joanne Lew '99

Swinging is highly effective in helping persons with ARMD learn to focus on the details of an object or figure by providing them with the conscious experience of the illusion that objects move when we move the head or body. It is also very helpful in improving coordination and balance.

A VARIATION OF SWINGING - FOCUS ON YOUR THUMB

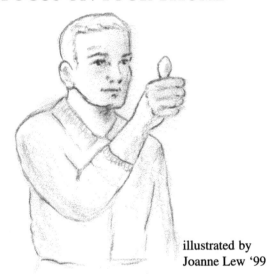

illustrated by
Joanne Lew '99

Focusing on your thumb while swinging is one of the most effective ways to train your eyes to see objects against a background. This exercise must be tried before its power can be experienced.

Exercise and Relax your Eyes

Sunning

Sunning is an exercise that is very soothing and easy to do. It is best done out of doors on a sunny day, but it can be done on a cloudy day outside or even while looking out a window. Sunning helps to rebuild the retina while it improves your psychological and emotional state. It also accustoms the eye to light and reduces photosensitivity. Some experts advise sunning with open eyes.

> *I do not advise this under any circumstances.*

Sunning should be done with firmly closed eyes. Then, while facing the sun, slowly turn your head from side to side. As you turn your head you will see the image of the sun move across your closed eyelids. It is probably best to do this exercise in the early morning with the rising sun or in the evening when the sun is setting. you should avoid the hours between 11:00a.m. and 2:00p.m. when the sun is at its brightest. Sunning should always be followed by a brief period of palming.

Sunning should be approached gently at first. Build to a comfortable level until you are doing it twice daily for ten minutes at a time. It is possible that at some point vivid 'after-images' will be produced by sunning. This is not a problem. The images can provide a strong focus for the attention and be very relaxing, but palming should be continued until the images have entirely disappeared and the field has returned to normal.

Slow and Rapid Blinking

This is a simple way to quickly relax your eyes anywhere, any time. It increases the production of tears, and tears deliver nutrients as well as moisture to the eye. Both are needed for good sight. Relax by focusing on your breath. Blink freely and often. Occasionally squeeze your eyes shut for a few seconds. This allows them to rest and shift focus. Alternate your rhythm of blinking so that you do it slowly and rapidly.

Squeeze blinking helps you produce tears whenever you need them to lubricate your eyes as well as bathing your eyes in nutrients. Squeeze your eyes shut for the count of three. Open your eyes wide. Relax the eyes and blink a few times.

Acupressure

Acupressure is a form of increasing the energy flow to the inner eye by applying light pressure and finger massage to certain points around the periphery of the eye. It can be done before or after palming. You will find these exercises very soothing and pleasant. There are many variations of this approach, but I am going to make it simple for you to learn and remember, in the hope that you do this often.

The following suggestions are taken from the work of Deborah Banker MD, an ophthalmologist who practices in Malibu, California. She offers a comprehensive and holistic approach to treating eye disease. She recom-

THE MAIN PRESSURE POINTS
AROUND THE EYE

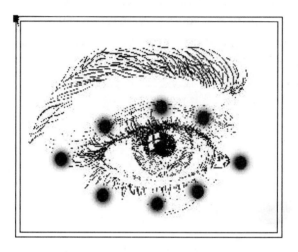

It is quite easy to touch upon all the major pressure points of the eye when you follow the three simple steps for massaging the bony area around the eye socket.

Massage:

1. the inner corners with your thumb
2. under the eyebrows with the side of your index finger
3. under the eye with your thumb or index finger pad

mends regular daily massage of the bony ridge around the eye as well as the entire face and head as a way to quickly brighten the vision. It is not so important to know where the pressure points are located exactly because they will be included in any kind of facial, head, and neck massage. The idea is to begin with a massage around the eye socket, move outward in ever widening circles to the rest of the face and neck, and then massage the scalp and back of the head and neck.

The first massage requires stimulating the bony ridge around the eye socket. There are three finger positions that make this easy and pleasant to do. You can use a little bland massage oil, or even olive oil, taking care not to get any in the eye.

> First: Massage the points at the inner corners of your eyes with your thumbs. Be sure your hands are clean and your nails are short.

> Second: Place your thumbs at the outer corners of your eyes and lightly massage along your eyebrows with the sides of your index fingers.

> Third: Using the pads of your index fingers or thumbs, gently press along the lower circle of bones under your eyes, from the outer corner to the inner, in a motion that continues the second step above. Because this tissue is very delicate, you may not want to stretch it with massage.

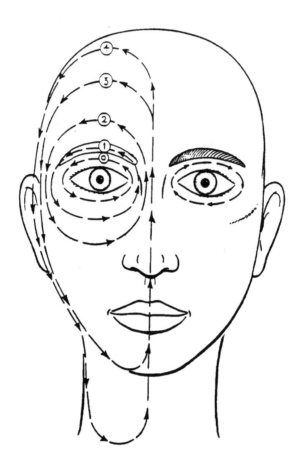

Continue to massage around your eye in ever-widening concentric circles until you have massaged your whole face and neck area.

Massage Your Whole Head

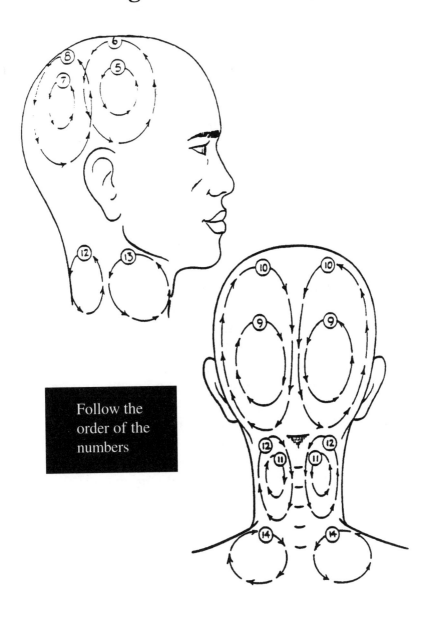

Follow the order of the numbers

Exercise and Relax your Eyes

Then, in the same basic direction, move over your whole eye area, and eventually your whole face in ever widening, concentric motions. Continue until you have included your hairline, the area in front of your ears, and your neck in these sweeping circles.

Finally, using your fingers like claws, sweep through your hair and scalp and back of the neck in circular motions. This will most likely feel very good and invigorating. You might ask a partner or friend to do this last step for you, if your range of motion in your arms is limited.

What to Expect

> Peter Manfield states: I have no doubt that a successful solution to the problem of ARMD will only be found by a holistic approach which addresses the physical, emotional, dynamic and mental aspects of the person's health. This will obviously include working directly on the vision and so far, the Bates approach with the modifications I have described, is an excellent way to bring about real improvement, with no pain, no danger - not even very much effort - just a lot of fun.

Hopefully your eye exercises and relaxation feel so good that you will do them without expectation of results. Most of my patients tell me that, once they begin these techniques, they feel so right that they have little trouble sticking to a regimen. I also recognize that persons with ARMD are apt to feel anxious about preserving and improving their vision. The effect of the vision therapy is like the effect of the relaxation response. It is a form of training, done in a relaxed state, that has a 'payoff' under stressful conditions. In terms of vision, stressful condition can include times of emotional tension as well as attempts to see things beyond one's range of vision. You may find that reading simply becomes easier. Often patients tell me that when they are reading something that was formerly difficult, they may 'freeze' up with the sudden awareness that they are seeing better, and then the letters blur again. This is a time to palm and blink. Many people report having flashes of extra clear vision at random times. These little 'gifts' show you that your vision is improving even if this does not show up on your next eye exam.

Trust yourself!

Checklist for Step Five

√   Learn to Palm, and do it daily.

√   Begin to swing every day.

√   Use Rapid Blinking to relax your eyes.

√   Find the Acupressure points around your eyes.

√   Combine these steps with the six ways to relax.

♦   Abdominal Breathing
♦   Affirmation
♦   Meditation
♦   Relax the Body
♦   Relax the Mind
♦   Breathe Consciously

Step 6 — Feed Your Macula for Better Sight

In the first chapter I attempted to give you a picture of the physiology of the eye and how macular degeneration affects the eye. I am now going to explain this in more detail in order to help you understand some of the nutritional recommendations I will make in this and the following chapters. First of all, the complete name of the macula is the macula lutea. This means yellow spot, and it is a bright yellow spot, about two millimeters in diameter in the center of the retina, which is about 20 mm in diameter itself. The macula is like a bull's eye that has the job of providing central vision and color vision.

If you have ever had a suntan, or if you have freckles or moles, you have seen evidence of the effect of melanin in your skin. Melanin is a pigment in the skin; the amount you have is genetically determined. Dark skinned people have an abundance of melanin while pale people have little. The purpose of melanin is to protect your skin from the harmful effects, or burn, from the sun. Similarly, there is a pigment in the eye that serves the same purpose. This is called the xanthophyll pigment. Its two forms are lutein and zeaxanthin. These yellow pigments are actually hidden in leafy green vegetables. When the leaves turn yellow or orange in autumn, they are 'revealing' the xanthophyll pigment that was obscured by chlorophyll. Certain green vegetables also turn yellow if allowed to age. Perhaps you have seen a nice fresh bunch of kale turn yellow in your vegetable bin.

Eat Colorful Foods to Enhance Your Eye Pigment

The job of these pigments is to absorb the blue rays of sunlight so that they do not burn the delicate tissues of the retina. While we are given a fairly good supply of them as children, most of us begin to lose xanthophyll pigments as early as the twenties or thirties. Daily consumption of leafy green vegetables, notably spinach, kale, mustard and collard greens keeps our eyes supplied with xanthophyll pigments. It is now understood that eating these foods is more significant for macular health than is the consumption of beta carotenes.

The good news is that research has shown that eating food rich in the xanthophyll pigments immediately increases the amount measurable in your blood, and soon after, the amount seen in the macula of the eye. The amount in the macula is measured by macula pigment density. Pigment in macula correlates to the health of the macula. Diminishing color vision occurs when the pigment density decreases. This is one of the early signs of ARMD. Because smoking seriously reduces both xanthophyll pigment levels in the blood as well as the pigment density of the macula, it is imperative to stop smoking now if you hope to heal your eye disease. There has been a lot of scientific documentation about the relationship between ARMD and smoking. Smoking is associated with a six fold increase in the likelihood of developing the condition. Second-hand smoke has also been implicated in ARMD developing in spouses of smokers.

Two Types Of Pigment

Lutein and zeaxanthin are the names of the specific carotenes required by the macula. The beta carotenes, which are more familiar to the American public, are found in carrots, squash, and sweet potatoes, and a host of other root and tuberous vegetables as well as fruit. Just about any richly colored produce is a source of beta carotene. While these foods and their nutrients are vital for overall health, including protection from cancer, it seems that the carotenes lutein and zeaxanthin are the most important for eye health. Lutein and zeaxanthin have been found to be present in abundance in just a few specific foods. These are, in the order of the amount of lutein and zeaxanthin they contain:

Kale	Cooked broccoli	*Best*
Spinach	Green peas	*Foods*
Parsley – fresh	Pumpkin	*for your*
Collard greens	Brussels sprouts	*Eyes!*
Mustard Greens	Corn	

Feed Your Macula

When these foods are eaten, lutein and zeaxanthin are deposited in the lungs, and the lens and macula of the eye. The fact that they are deposited in the lens demonstrates their ability to protect against and reverse cataracts. Since many people have both ARMD and cataracts, or a tendency to cataracts, these powerful nutrients are a double boon. Grace Halloran, author of *Amazing Grace*, and a world-renowned vision instructor, observes that when there is an insufficient supply of lutein and Zeaxanthin, the body will deposit available amounts in the lungs and starve the eyes since the lungs are more important for sustaining life than are the eyes. This sparing by the body is completely unnecessary when enough lutein-containing food is consumed on a daily basis. I say, let the eyes have it! Eat enough of it.

Lutein and zeaxanthin are the dominant pigments in the retina. It is postulated that they filter out harmful blue light rays from the rays that reach the retina. Other light, notably ultraviolet light, is filtered out by the cornea and lens. A retina dense with lutein and zeaxanthin can better handle this task. The results of supplementation and consumption of more lutein and zeaxanthin is enhanced visual sensitivity, sharper color vision, less eye fatigue and strain, better contrast, and better night vision.

Research On Lutein And Zeaxanthin

Many studies have been done in an attempt to show the relationship between the consumption of lutein and zeaxanthin and the development of macular degeneration. The most conclusive thing that has been proven is that there is a direct correlation between eating lutein-rich foods and macular health. One study looked at the past dietary habits of people who ate a lot food containing lutein and zeaxanthin as well as those who did not and attempted to determine the impact of the diets of each group on the development of ARMD. The outcome of this study was most interesting. It determined that individuals who had a history of consuming lots of foods with lutein and zeaxanthin reduced their likelihood of developing ARMD by 86%.

The second study divided a large group of people into two groups and gave each group a different diet. The first group ate a lot of foods with lutein and zeaxanthin, and the second group at very little of those foods. This study was used to measure whether eating foods rich in lutein and zeaxanthin produced elevated levels of these carotenoids in their bloodstream. It did.

> **It was also demonstrated that people who ate the lutein-rich diet had a measurably thicker macula.**

A report in the Journal of the American Medical Association (JAMA) found that adults who consume the equivalent of five servings of spinach per week reduce their risk of developing macular degeneration by 57%. How does this affect those who already have the condition? Although we cannot answer this for certain, it seems reasonable to assume that these nutrients have a huge impact on the health and functioning of the retina. Therefore, it seems prudent to add them in quantity to your diet.

Following are four statements that can be made about the relationship between dietary lutein and zeaxanthin and macular degeneration:

1. Eating foods with lutein and zeaxanthin in creases the amount of lutein and zeaxanthin available to the body.

2. Eating foods with lutein and zeaxanthin thickens macular pigment.

3. An increase in macular pigment reduces the risk of ARMD.

4. Eating foods with lutein and zeaxanthin *reduces the chance of developing ARMD.*

Remember These Facts!!

If you already have ARMD, the addition of these nutrients will help stabilize your vision at its present level. It may help you regain some of the sight you have lost by optimizing the functioning of the healthy parts of your macula, including cells that have been nutritionally starved for decades. It will also set the stage to enhance the effectiveness of any of the other techniques I will describe in the final chapters of the book. Your success with them is highly dependent on improving not only your overall health, but the health of your eye tissues and cells.

A Green Diet

I realize that the typical American diet contains very little of the foods now considered vital to eye as well as overall health. No fast food I have ever seen contains leafy green vegetables or broccoli. In fact, aside from anemic lettuce and tomatoes, fast food contains very little in the way of vegetables. Spinach can be ordered at most restaurants, but the other types of vegetables are rarely seen on a menu. Once again, I need to emphasize the benefits of home cooking. Eating at least one home cooked meal each day is the only way to ensure consuming the necessary quantities of greens. In addition to eating one home cooked meal, I urge you to lunch on leftovers from this meal. Adopt the habit of eating soup for breakfast if it agrees with you. With a little discipline, you can easily consume three to five servings of vegetables and fruit by lunch time.

Leafy Greens Rule

You will need to become creative at preparing daily

servings of green leafy vegetables if you wish to improve the health of your eyes. Greens cooked with garlic and onions often appeal more readily than those prepared plain. However, remember to avoid cooking methods that kill the vital carotenes. Do not fry greens. Sauté, steam, or gently bake them in their own juices. Although they may not win popularity contests at the dinner table, all members of your family will benefit from this change in your diet.

Now that I have motivated you to eat food for your macula, I want to emphasize the importance of being able to digest it. Many people, particularly the aged and those with chronic illness, have impaired bowel function. This means that nutrients from food pass through without being absorbed in your bloodstream and circulated to the organs and tissues that need them so desperately. One way to support the digestion of carotene is to take your supplements with food since they require fat enzymes to break them down. Alternatively you can take digestive enzymes with them. Lutein and zeaxanthin should not be taken at the same time as other beta carotene supplements since the absorption of the other types of carotenes can interfere with the absorption of lutein and zeaxanthin.

Detoxify

A toxic condition results from the build-up of cellular waste in the body. This is exactly what causes macular degeneration. Therefore, it is reasonable to assume that waste clearing processes have slowed down or ceased throughout your system. Traditional means of detoxifying included enemas, saunas, fasting and the use of colonics to rid the body of waste through the normal channels of the colon and skin. Fortunately, research into the dynamics of detoxification have resulted in the production of organ stimulating supplements that are highly effective in ridding the body of wastes and setting the stage for optimal nutrition.

Supplement With Lutein

Since the recent discovery of the importance of lutein and zeaxanthin on macular health, many nutritional supplements containing them have been formulated. I urge everyone with ARMD to include these supplements in their daily diet in addition to the dietary addition of lutein-rich food. Food is still the best source of lutein, and supplements do just that – add to the available level of nutrients. Lutein is found in abundance in marigolds and sunflowers and protects these plants from sun damage. These flowers provide the source of the lutein used in supplements. Because zeaxanthin is made from lutein, only a small amount is needed as a supplement. It is advisable to take supplements containing lutein at times other than the time you take beta carotene supplements to enhance absorption of the lutein. However, when eating foods rich in lutein and zeaxanthin, it is fine to mix your greens with squash and tomatoes because, when they are absorbed from food, all the beta carotenes work well together.

Feed Your Macula

Lutein supplementation should be between 100 and 200 milligrams daily. For my patients, I recommend a product called Pure Focus™.

This is a spray that is taken orally three times per day. It contains 200 milligrams of lutein, 8 milligrams of zinc, and 750 milligrams of bilberry, an herb that is vital to good vision. In addition, Pure Focus™ has 320 milligrams of vimpocetine, and 300 IUs of Vitamin E. Vimpocetine is derived from periwinkle seed. When 100 patients with arteriosclerosis and eye disorders were treated with vimpocetine, 88 percent had an increase in retinal circulation and improved vision. This formula:

- increases blood flow to the brain
- improves the utilization of oxygen and glucose
- increases the turnover of norepinephrine and serotonin.

The advantage of using a spray form of nutrient is that the nutrients are absorbed immediately into the bloodstream when the liquid is left in the mouth for two minutes. This means that even those with poor digestion can receive the full impact of the nutrients.

How soon should you expect to notice results from adding lutein-rich foods and supplements to your diet? Many people will notice improvement after six to eight weeks. Some will see improvement earlier, while others may not notice much improvement for ninety days or so. The important thing is to begin and maintain. Do not stop after just a short time because there are no dramatic changes. Remember: your condition probably began developing decades before you noticed it. It is normal for it to take a while to respond to these health-enhancing measures. You cannot lose because these foods and supplements are the same as those recommended to protect against cancer and heart disease. They are bound to enhance your overall vitality significantly. Please read on to see what else you can do to heal your vision!

Checklist For Step Six

√ Memorize the list of foods that feed
    your eyes

√ Introduce one new food from this list
    per week into your diet

√ Order Pure Focus™ and give it a try.

(See Resources for ordering information)

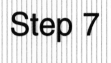 **Step 7** Supplement
Your Diet

Do You Need Supplements?

Many people insist that they can get all their nutrients from food. "If God wanted me to take vitamins, He would have made a vitamin pill" typifies their thinking. The American public has long been told by the medical profession that all the nutrients they require are available through a 'good diet' and that vitamins do nothing but create expensive urine. The truth is that most doctors know very little about nutrition. Virtually nothing is taught in medical schools. At least at the time I attended, the emphasis was on curing disease not preventing it. While pharmaceutical companies were loud and clear in promoting the benefits of drugs of every type, we never heard from representatives of vitamin companies. In fact we were taught to regard the whole health food and supplement field with scorn. As a young medical student, however, I had the unique opportunity of doing a three month nutritional rotation at the University of California at Davis. Here I learned about the benefits of supplementing the diet.

111

Supplement Your Diet

I now know that pharmaceutical companies have an interest in making people take medicine and in encouraging doctors to write prescriptions. They are among the most profitable industries in our country. On the other hand, if we were taught to focus on prevention and health maintenance, including the use of vitamins and minerals, pharmaceutical companies might not be so profitable. It seems to me that it is a lot safer to have some Vitamin C wash out of your system in your urine than to accept the side effects of virtually all prescription drugs.

Another important factor in the campaign against supplements is that we really don't know how much of any nutrient people need to be healthy in our current environment. The government has established something called the RDA – Recommended Daily Allowance of the major vitamins and minerals. These amounts, however, were developed by determining how much of the substance was needed to prevent disease. The RDA for Vitamin C, for example, is the amount required to prevent scurvy. These studies were done on young healthy persons many years ago before we had to contend with our denatured food and environmental toxins. In a diseased state the requirements of vitamins are increased. The damaged or injured cells are trying to repair themselves and need more nutrients.

A third reason why supplements have been controversial is that, until recent decades, there were no studies that demonstrated how valuable they were. Pharmaceutical companies had no financial incentive to perform studies on a product that they could not patent. Doctors believe in studies because they are scientifically acceptable. So now we have studies showing the role of Vitamin C in protecting against many diseases; Vitamin E protecting against heart disease, and an herb, St. John's Wort, helping with depression.

I firmly believe that it is prudent for almost everyone to supplement their diet. It certainly is necessary for persons who are aged, who have a chronic illness, who are exposed to toxins or other environmental hazards, who handle stressful situations poorly, and who have a family history of heart disease, cancer, or diabetes. I add serious eye disease to this list, of course. This is why I can safely say that virtually everyone needs to take supplements. The amount and particular mix of supplements for an individual depends on age, overall health, family history, and any early signs of degenerative disease.

Supplement Dosage

I have just explained how the RDA dosage of supplements is determined. This level of nutritional supplements is too low for almost everyone. Since you will be using nutrients like medicine, you need to take larger amounts of the nutrients recommended in this chapter. After explaining each nutrient, I will share with you a formula that contains an adequate amount of each one. Taking this formula, or a similar one, will ensure that you receive sufficient amounts of every indicated vitamin and mineral discussed. You could take more of some of the nutrients, but you would need to buy extra bottles of pills and capsules.

Anti-Oxidants and Free Radicals

Many of the supplements that I want you to take are called anti-oxidants. They counteract the damage done to your body by free radicals. All of this is explained in the next section. I want to emphasize that taking these supplements is critical if you hope to improve you eye disease. They will boost your overall health enormously in the process. One caveat is that you need to be able to assimilate them. Re-read the section in the previous chapter about detoxifying your body.

Many people find that they are more motivated to take anti-oxidants once they know more about how free radicals are created. Body cells use oxygen to break down proteins, carbohydrates, and fats and convert them to forms of energy the cells can use for metabolic processes. This breaking down of oxygen produces free radicals. Free radicals are atoms with an extra electron in their cell. This makes them unstable and highly attracted to bonding with other molecules. However, some of the bonds they make may result in molecules that are destructive to cells and to the DNA in cells. The effects of this can be as minimal as wrinkles or as harmful as cancer. Anti-oxidants are like scavengers for free radicals. They nip them in the bud so to speak before they can do any damage. That is why they are also called 'free radical scavengers.' Because our metabolic processes are ongoing, every day, we need to replenish our free radical scavengers by consuming foods and supplements with anti-oxidant properties on a daily basis.

Now I am going to list each anti-oxidant vitamin and mineral that I want you to include in your supplementation plan. These will be in addition to eating foods with lutein and zeaxanthin and taking these as supplements as discussed in the last chapter. I also want you to read the next chapter and learn about the herbs that I want you to include as supplements. This means that you will be taking a lot of supplements for a long time. It will cost you money out of pocket. But remember, you have a serious disease that threatens to interfere with your independence and mobility in a serious way. Further, that condition is probably only a sign that overall health status is compromised. There are no medical miracles for ARMD. If you do nothing, your vision will probably deteriorate. What have you got to lose?

Vitamins

Vitamin A

This was the first vitamin discovered; hence its name. It is also called retinol because of its importance in vision, especially in night vision. It is also very important in the formation and maintenance of healthy skin, internal tissues, bone, and hair. Pre-formed Vitamin A is available in cod liver oil and in the livers of animals as well as dairy products. Vitamin A is fat soluble, and it is stored in the liver, kidneys, lungs, eyes, and fat tissue. It needs

Supplement Your Diet

Vitamin E to expedite absorption and Zinc in order to release it for use in the body. Provitamin A as beta-carotene is available from orange, yellow, and green vegetables and fruits.

A great deal has been written warning people not to take too much Vitamin A. Indeed, because this nutrient is stored in the body, it is possible to develop Vitamin A toxicity characterized by dry skin, nausea, and loss of appetite. Pregnant women should not consume large doses of Vitamin A. Many people like to avoid the Vitamin A toxicity problem by taking all their Vitamin A as beta-carotene, a substance that converts to Vitamin A on an as-needed basis. This is a fine idea – as long as you have a normal thyroid. Some researches think that a large number of people cannot convert beta carotene to Vitamin A because they have hypothyroidism, the term for an underactive thyroid. Still other scientists think that a large percentage of people with ARMD have hypothyroidism, regardless of whether it has shown up on tests or not. Additionally, zinc is needed to use Vitamin A and many prescription drugs deplete Zinc. Since night blindness is one of the first indications that ARMD or another serious eye condition is developing, I have come to regard Vitamin A deficiency as prime in creating the conditions for ARMD. Therefore, taking Vitamin A is essential in your program to reverse ARMD.

Beta Carotene

This nutrient, found abundantly in foods, is called a Vitamin A precursor. This means that it converts readily to Vitamin A in the body as the body's requirement for Vitamin A demands it. It is water-soluble, unlike Vitamin A which is stored in fat tissue.

In the last chapter, you were introduced to specific foods that contain types of beta-carotene known to support the health of the macula. When you add these to your diet regularly, you are adding a good source of beta-carotene from food.

Vitamin C

Vitamin C is perhaps the most accepted and well-known of the supplements. So much has been learned about the protective benefits of supplementing the diet above the 60mg RDA that the federal government is in the process of revising the RDA upwards. As a balance to this, recent studies have shown that the megadoses of Vitamin C recommended over the past years by specialists in natural health are unwarranted. Dr. Andrew Weil, an author, and nutritional expert, who formerly recommended 1000 to 5000mg (1-5 grams) per day of Vitamin C has now revised his maintenance dose recommendation to 250-500mg per day.

Human beings are not able to create Vitamin C as are most other animals. It must be obtained on a daily basis from food and supplements. A small amount is stored in areas of high metabolism in the body, including the eyes. Vitamin C is easily absorbed and easily excreted. Whatever is taken in lasts only a few hours. Therefore, frequent snacking on citrus fruit as well as taking supplements in divided doses is recommended.

Supplement Your Diet

Vitamin C's main function in the body is to strengthen collagen, the fibrous material in the skeleton and surrounding each cell. It also aids in the production of thyroid hormone and in lowering cholesterol. Because it strengthens the cell walls, it is an anti-oxidant par excellence since strong cell walls prevent damage from free radicals.

Vitamin C, as a supplement, comes in many forms including tablets, capsules, powders, effervescents, and chewable tablets. When combined with calcium and magnesium and/or potassium, it can be soothing to the stomach rather than irritating. Diarrhea is a result of excess Vitamin C consumption. It is easily handled by reducing your dosage.

Vitamin E

The food sources of Vitamin E are the oils in all grains, seeds, and nuts. Wheat germ oil is an especially rich source. Vitamin E works to protect and enhance the cell membranes of the skin, eyes, and liver from free radical damage. It is a fat-soluble vitamin, like Vitamin A, and is absorbed from the intestines and stored in the liver and fatty tissue, heart, and muscles. It is not as stable in the body as Vitamin A, and more is lost through excretion. When taken as a supplement, the best form of Vitamin E is mixed tocopherols. It was formerly believed that d-alpha tocopherol was the best form, but that view has been modified. Much less valuable is dl-alpha tocopherol. I do not recommend this synthetic form. Magnesium levels (see below) need to be adequate for the **most efficient use of Vitamin E.**

118

Minerals

Chromium

Although chromium is needed in minute quantity in the body, a deficiency may lead to serious metabolic disorders. Diabetics almost all show a deficiency of Chromium, and it plays an important role in blood vessel health. Our chronic deficiency is most likely due to depleted soil and over-processed food. Fortunately most multiple vitamin and mineral supplements contain the amount needed on a daily basis.

Selenium

Selenium is another micro nutrient whose deficiency is associated with depleted soils. The amount of selenium in the soil and water of an area can vary greatly. However, conservative supplementation of the diet is not thought to produce any toxicity. The lens of cataract patients have shown far lower levels of selenium than are present in healthy tissue. This produces a strong association between eye health and selenium levels. Selenium is found in a wide variety of foods, and a diet rich in natural foods from selenium-rich soil may provide adequate amounts. However, if you have a serious disease, I would venture a guess that your intake of Selenium is inadequate.

Selenium needs Vitamin E to perform its anti-oxidant functions. I recommend that you take these two nutrients together. It can be inhibited by Vitamin C, which should be taken at a different time of the day.

Supplement Your Diet

Zinc

Zinc is another mineral diminished due to poor soil. An added problem in obtaining adequate zinc is that meat and animal foods are the most abundant sources. We are recommending a diet high in produce and grains and lower in animal products. Yet Zinc is needed by virtually all the tissues in the body. When it is stored, the retina contains the second highest concentration (male sexual organs the highest).Zinc is also necessary to transport Vitamin A to the eye and to combat free radical damage.

As important as it is to obtain adequate amounts of zinc, by far the greater problem is how easily it is lost or depleted. It can be sweated away during exercise, burned up during stress, and this includes stress from surgery or injury or illness as well as emotional stress. For elders, a big problem is that zinc is depleted in metabolizing many commonly prescribed drugs for hypertension, high cholesterol, and many other conditions.

There are two other supplements that are very valuable anti-oxidants. The first is Gamma linolenic acid. Good sources for this are evening primrose, black currant seed, and black walnut oil. It is very important for people with low thyroid function to supplement with this nutrient. Its usefulness in wet ARMD is unparalleled since its main work in the body is to heal and support blood vessel walls. The other nutrient is Lecithin. Lecithin helps lower cholesterol levels and helps the eye to see, thereby revealing the relationship between the eye and the liver that is understood so well in Chinese medicine. Lecithin can be taken in capsule or granule form. Granules can be sprinkled on cereal.

And, finally, I need to mention Taurine. Taurine is a sulfur-containing amino acid which is found naturally in egg whites and meat and fish proteins. It has a protective effect on the heart and blood vessels, but, most importantly, it is found in the retina. Adequate levels of zinc are needed to aid taurine in its role of cellular metabolism and nerve impulse generation. Daily supplementation at 500 mg of taurine is advised.

How to Get All your Vitamins and Minerals

Taking a lot of pills on a daily basis, even for the most determined and motivated person can be a problem. Multi vitamin and mineral pills solve this problem to some extent, but their ingredients may not be adequate for your needs. That is why I worked with a company to develop what I believe to be the most complete supplement for persons with macular degeneration. The formula I developed is the Macular Degeneration Nutritional Formula available from Nutritional Research LLC in Carson City, Nevada. This product contains 29 ingredients, including the anti-oxidants mentioned above, lutein, and the herbs I will describe in the next chapter. This product is made from the freshest natural extracts. No artificial additives, preservatives, corn, wheat, yeast or soy or dairy products are used in the manufacturing. The nutrients are put into capsules so patients who have difficulty swallowing can open the capsule and mix the contents into fruit juice or sprinkle it on cereal. There are many other formulas on the market, and you may choose to purchase any one. Just be sure that your bases are covered in terms of the anti-oxidant power available in any given brand. You will probably need to supplement with individual nutrients in the first three months regardless of what brand you choose since the therapeutic doses are too high to be carried in a single pill. This has it all! You will see several ingredients listed that I did not cover in this chapter. Be assured that they are very important for total eye health.

Following is a list of the ingredients in the macular degeneration formulation that I recommend. For those patients who do not want to buy an extra product (i.e. **Pure Focus**™), and wish to take all their nutrients from this formula, it contains a baseline level of lutein, vitamin E, and zeaxanthin.

Six capsules of the
Macular Degeneration Nutritional Formula
available from Nutritional Research LLC contain

Vitamin A (palmitate) 5000 IU
Beta Carotene 10,000 IU, (providing Zeaxanthin 18 mcg,
alpha carotene 90 mcg, cryptoxanthin 22 mcg)
Vitamin B-1 (Thiamine)25 mg
Vitamin B-2 (Riboflavin) 25 mg
Vitamin B-3 (Niacinamide) 50 mg
Vitamin B-3 (Niacin) 10 mg
Vitamin B-5 (Pantothenic Acid) 100 mg
Vitamin B-6 (Pyridoxine HCI) 25 mg
Folio Acid 200 mcg
Vitamin B-12 100 mcg
Vitamin C 500 mg
Vitamin E (d-alpha Tocopherol) 200 IU
N-Acetyl L-Cysteine 200 mg
Bilberry Extract 40 mg
Ginkgo Biloba Extract 40 mg
Quercitin Bioflavonoid 50 mg
L-Taurine 400 mg
Calcium (Citrate) 100 mg
Magnesium (Citrate) 200 mg
Copper (Sebecate) 3 mg
Selenium (Selenomethionine) 200 mcg
Zinc (Picolinate) 20 mg
L-Glutathione 25 mg
Manganese 3 mg
Rutin 15 mg
Hesperidin 10 mg
Lycopene 1 mg
Lutein 10 mg

Supplement Your Diet

You can see how comprehensive this formula is. Although you do need to take six capsules in divided doses, you will be getting virtually all the nutrients needed for your eye health. Of course your overall health will improve immensely when you begin to supplement your diet at this level. Taking supplements and improving your diet are two of the most important ways anyone can improve overall health.Congratualtions on taking care of yourself!

Checklist for Step Seven

√ Read the labels on your vitamins and list
　　all those you are now taking

√ Compare this list to the Macular Degenera
　　tion Formula

√ Order the Macular Degeneration Formula
　　or purchase individual supplements
　　for your eye health
　　(See Resources)

Supplement Your Diet

Step 8 | Three Herbs for Your Vision

This is the third chapter discussing substances you need to add to your diet in order to heal your vision. In Step Six I urged you to take a supplement that contains a significant amount of lutein and zeaxanthin. Step Seven was an overview of the vitamins and minerals you need. Step Eight discusses the three herbs known for centuries to have a toning and healing effect on the eyes. You may be able to find many of these in the same supplements you take for your overall eye health. If you do, that is great. Otherwise, you may need to buy separate bottles of capsules and tablets in order to ensure that you have your bases covered. Step Twelve will help you formulate your personal plan for implementing the steps in this book.

Herbal medicine is gaining respectability among the American public and even among conventional doctors. The use of herbs in Chinese medicine is now an accepted part of treatment by an acupuncturist. Often this treatment is available in HMOs or as part of conventional doctors' practices. It is taking longer for our own western herbs to gain acceptance. Yet these are also powerful and effective sources of health maintenance and healing. Since treatment with western herbs is usually a self care activity, people need to become educated about the various herbs and what they can do to strengthen and heal the body and the mind.

Recently, St. John's Wort has received a lot of interest and scientific investigation for its ability to help people cope with depression and anxiety. Once scientists demonstrated its effectiveness, it became the front line of medicine even for conventionally trained doctors. Many are now willing to recommend it before writing a prescription for Prozac or another anti-depressant. I don't know when eye doctors, as a group, will begin to recognize the value of herbs for the eyes. I have found them to be very valuable as part of a mix of treatments I suggest to my patients who have ARMD, glaucoma, and cataracts. You can safely begin taking these herbs as soon as you have read about this step.

What Are Herbs?

Herbs are plants that are used for medicinal or culinary purposes. We are all familiar with mint and rosemary. Some people like to cultivate basil, marjoram, thyme or chives to enhance the flavor of food. While culinary herbs have medicinal properties, these properties are barely noticed in the quantities we take as part of the diet. However, you might notice that drinking mint tea after a meal aids your digestion or that eating parsley causes you to urinate more. Some naturalists maintain that every plant on earth has healing properties, but that we do not understand them all. One thing is certain – there are numerous herbs, and they work for all sorts of human ills.

The medicinal part of a plant can be the leaves, flowers, fruit, roots, or bark. Herbs that use the root or bark are usually, but not always, stronger and less tasty than those made from leaves and flowers. Some herbs are organically grown, and, of course, if you can find an herbal supplement made from an organic plant, choose it over another one. Wildcrafting is a term used to describe how herbs are obtained. This means that someone found them growing in nature and picked them. It implies that there are no pesticides or chemicals used in their production, but since the definition of 'organic' is strictly regulated in many states, wildcrafted herbs cannot claim to be organic. They are an excellent choice, however. Some herbal formulas use only the active ingredient of an herb, the one alkaloid thought to be responsible for the herb's healing powers. This is actually not a good idea since we really do not know if an herb acts only through its 'active' ingredient or through the synergy of all its living components. It is usually best to use the full plant part.

How to Take Herbs

Herbal supplements come in liquid and dry form. The liquid form is a tincture, made from a concentration of the herbs juices preserved in a medium such as alcohol, water, or glycerin. Dried herbs come in capsules or tablets. Tinctures offer the advantage of being easy to take and readily absorbed through the mucous membranes of the mouth. For this reason, I prefer tinctures for my patients. Capsules are the next best in that the herbal matter is readily available once the gelatin capsule has dissolved. Tablets are my least favorite since they are hard to break down in the digestive tract. If you are getting some of your herbal requirements in a multi nutrient tablet, consider taking the balance as a tincture. Herbs are food and can be taken with meals or separately if they cause you no gastric distress.

Usually a course of herbal treatment should be maintained for at least thirty to ninety days. For ARMD patients, because of the slow progression of the disease, you may have to take herbs for as long as six months before you notice any improvement in your vision. The herbs I will discuss in this chapter will help slow down the progression of your disease and you should continue taking them even if you are not sure they are helping your vision. Some herbalists recommend taking herbs six days of each week to give your body a chance to respond on the seventh day.

Bilberry

During World War II, British fighter pilots are said to have eaten bilberry preserves in order to improve their night vision. This practice probably grew out of folklore in Europe that considered bilberry to enhance sight. Bilberry is a plant known as Vaccinium myrtillus. The medicinal part is the fruit or berries, and closely resembles American huckleberries. The plant grows in Europe and the Rocky Mountain region.

Bilberry acts as an anti-oxidant in combating free radical damage and stabilizing collagen as well as strengthening capillaries. Although the leaves of the plant are poisonous, the fruit has no adverse reaction, even when taken in large amounts. In several studies, patients with various eye disorders ranging from myopia to macular degeneration, showed improvement in their vision a short time after taking bilberry. In another study, bilberry plus Vitamin E stopped the progression of cataracts in 97% of the patients on the regimen. Daily supplementation with Bilberry as it is included in a total eye formula is highly recommended.

Ginkgo biloba

This supplement is derived from the leaves of the Ginkgo biloba tree, one of the oldest plants on earth. Its age points to its application in many of the disorders associated with aging, among them senility and loss of memory. Ginkgo biloba improves circulation to the brain through a mild blood thinning effect. For this reason, it should never be used by anyone who is taking blood thinners. It is helpful in macular degeneration because, by stimulating the blood flow to the eye, waste material in the form of drusen can more easily be carried away. Grace Halloran, author of *Amazing Grace*, who works with visually impaired people in a comprehensive training program (see last chapter), states that several of her clients have had their drusen completely disappear. These were individuals of varying ages, who methodically developed and maintained a healing plan like the one I am suggesting in this book.

Ginkgo biloba also relieves depression and helps with hardening of the arteries (atherosclerosis). Because of its effect on the blood vessels of the eye, Ginkgo biloba is very important as a supplement for those with wet ARMD as well as for anyone with cerebral insufficiency syndrome which is lack of proper circulation to the brain.

Because of the extensive research done with this herb, it has been found that a preparation containing 24 percent ginkgosides is the most effective. When you purchase Ginkgo biloba, look for a brand that is made by a reputable herbal pharmacy and that contains this amount of its active ingredient. A dosage of 120mg per day is sufficient to obtain benefits from this marvelous substance. You may find this included in eye health formulas.

Eyebright

Eyebright or *Euphrasia officinalis* is an herb that has been used to help heal eye condition since early Greek times. There are references to it in Elizabethan literature. It is taken internally, either as an herbal tincture or cap-

sule or tablet, or as a homeopathic remedy. I will discuss
its homeopathic use in the chapter on homeopathy. Eye-
washes have been made from Eyebright also, but you are
advised not to make your own since it can be irritating.
Eyebright can be used as a soothing compress on the
closed eyes. To make a compress, use an eyebright tea
bag. They are available in most health food stores or
through www.nutritionalresearch.net. The tea bag can also
be used as a compress applied directly to the eye and the
"tea" can be consumed. Eyebright tea is usually not irritating to the eye. If you cannot locate tea bags then you
can use one teaspoon of powdered herb or open a capsule and add 1 cup boiling water. Allow the mixture to
cool and soak cotton balls or squares in it. Place these on
your eyes while you relax. This treatment can be used at
the same time you do sunning or palming exercises.

The medicinal parts of the plant are its flowers and
leaves. Its primary medicinal use has been to treat con-
junctivitis and eye strain. It has been found helpful in
light sensitivity as well as stinging and tearing eyes. In
folklore it was used to treat 'dim vision.' Herbalists believe that Eyebright acts to tonify the liver, and that this
explains its impact on the eyes – Chinese theory again.
To supplement with Eyebright, if taken internally, take
two capsules, about 450-500mg each, daily. If Eyebright
is included in any of your other supplement formulas,
you probably do not need to take an additional amount.

Three Herbs for Your Vision

The Power of Herbs

Nature provides us with virtually everything we need for healing. As we experience the negative impact of most pharmaceutical drugs, we will turn more and more often to the healing power of nature. Just because herbs are readily available does not mean that they are not powerful. I am thankful that these potent healing substances can be bought and used freely. I urge you to take the information in this chapter to heart and begin to use them. In the next section of the book, I will describe powerful and unique ways to treat ARMD. Use the wisdom of the last three steps to get your eyes ready to respond.

Checklist for Step Eight

√ Visit your library and browse through books on herbs.

√ Purchase some mild herbal tea and begin to enjoy a cup every day.

√ Visit your health food store and find supplements that contain:
- Bilberry
- Ginkgo biloba
- Eyebright

Three Herbs for Your Vision

	Chelation Therapy:
Step 9	Improve Circulation
	to Your Eye

With this chapter I will describe the first of three ways to treat ARMD that may be completely new to both you and your doctor. I recommend that my patients add one or more of these techniques to the rest of the steps I have described, in order to maximize their chances of reversing ARMD. You may wonder why I didn't just explain these in the beginning of the book and forget all that information about diet, exercise, stress management, and supplements. First, you must recognize that these three therapies: Chelation, Microcurrent Stimulation, and Homeopathy require your own natural vital force in order to work well. These are not drugs that you can take or operations you can undergo where you have no active part in your healing. On the contrary, for these methods to work as well as they can, you must be in the best possible health. The second reason why the first part of this book is so important is that your ARMD developed because you have some sort of systemic degeneration in progress, even if your ARMD is the only sign of it. Therefore, I have given you the tools to improve your underlying state of health. With optimal health, you can handle your ARMD much better on the emotional level and cope with vision changes and mobility issues much more successfully while you are waiting for improved vision. Finally, after the therapeutic segment of your healing program ends, you will need to be involved in a maintenance program to ensure that your new found visual gains are not lost due to poor lifestyle habits.

Chelation Therapy

Francis Gmys is a hard working farmer in Home, Pennsylvania. Besides being a very likeable and friendly person, he is my uncle. In 1983, Sonny (that is what everyone calls him) developed chest pains that were so debilitating he could not walk to the barn without many stops. He took nitroglycerine tablets all day long. When he consulted a doctor, he learned that he had 70% blockage in a cardiac artery and would need by-pass surgery in two years. Around this time he learned that several of his neighbors were undergoing chelation therapy for their heart conditions and other blood vessel problems. He joined the carpool of neighbors who went to Mount Pleasant for their weekly treatments. He says that far from unpleasant, he found the treatments very enjoyable. He saw people get stronger every week. There was always someone to talk to.

In all, Sonny had 46 chelation treatments. He had no more chest pain and was feeling great. Because of this, he made a mistake he still regrets. He got busy back at the farm and did not take his monthly maintenance treatments as the doctor strongly recommended. Three years later the chest pain was back. He took 10 treatments but they did not bring him the relief he experienced earlier. So he had the surgery and, "it did not help me at all." Now he is back to chelation and hopes to have the same outcome he first experienced. This time he will do the maintenance program!

The first technique I want to describe to you is called Chelation Therapy. Although you may never have heard of chelation, it has been employed by doctors in this country since about 1950, following its development in Germany in 1938. This is a treatment normally used to treat lead poisoning and even venomous snake bites in medicine. It was found, in the early years of its use, that chelation improved the heart disease of those who underwent it for other purposes. This prompted a number of physicians to begin using it for this purpose since it is known to flush plaque and toxic metals from bloodstream. For many, many individuals it has been an alternative to heart or vascular surgery.

In chelation therapy, about three grams of EDTA is used for each treatment. Although it has been approved to treat lead poisoning and some other conditions, it has not been approved for use in treating heart and vascular conditions. This does not mean that it is harmful or ineffective in these instances. Many drugs and devices are used in this way in the medical field. When doctors use chelation for purposes other than lead poisoning, they are using an approved substance, the synthetic amino acid EDTA (ethyl diamine tetra acetic acid) in a discretionary way. This is done frequently in medicine. One example familiar to us all is the use of aspirin, which is approved for the treatment of pain. Physicians routinely recommend it to thin the blood of persons with cardiovascular disease.

How is Chelation Administered?

A chelation treatment requires a visit to a doctor's office where a substance is infused into your veins through an IV for the purpose of helping your body rid itself of toxic heavy metals and excess minerals. Chelation requires a course of treatment of several sessions per week for several weeks or months. ACAM recommends that patients undergo 30 chelation treatments in order to obtain the optimum effect, and follow these with a maintenance dose once a month. Each session lasts two to four hours. The frequency of the treatments depends on the severity of the condition and the way that the body is handling the excretion of the minerals. During the course of treatment, the doctor will monitor the health of kidneys as well as other organs to ensure that no undue stress is placed on the body. There is almost no discomfort with chelation and the side effects, which are rare, are very minimal. Patients are instructed during this time in proper diet, stress management, and exercise regimens to support their overall recovery.

Chelation is administered by medical doctors (MDs) and Doctors of Osteopathy (DOs) who have been specially trained in this therapy and are accredited by the American College for the Advancement of Medicine (ACAM). This organization was founded in 1973 as a medical society to educate and update physicians on the latest in preventive and nutritional advances against disease. Although there may be other health practitioners who use chelation, I would strongly recommend that you work only with a doctor who is a member of ACAM. This means that he or she knows how to match the dose of EDTA to your particular condition and to monitor your overall health during the course of treatment. A list of doctors can be obtained by calling ACAM at (949) 583-7666 or visit their web page at www.acam.org.

> I have performed Chelation therapy, using EDTA and other nutrients, in my office for the past ten years. It has resulted in distinct visual changes such as improved acuity and color vision in many patients.
>
> Harold Byer, MD,
> Ophthalmologist,
> Fountainview, PA.

I want to emphasize that, in the more than 40 years it has been used in this country, only two deaths have occurred that can be attributed to chelation. These occurred in the fifties, when there was insufficient knowledge about drug dosage and administration. Conventional medicine has made much of these two deaths while they conveniently ignore the 100,000 deaths each year from prescription drugs

Chelation has been used very successfully to treat cardiovascular disease, diabetes, diabetic arterial disease, decreased mental functioning, intermittent claudication (leg pain on exercise), and a number of other conditions. Eye conditions such as glaucoma and cataracts have responded to chelation therapy. It has also been used to reverse macular degeneration since ARMD is caused, at least in part, by the blockage in the choroid capillaries which deliver blood to the macula.

In 1994, the Journal of the Advancement of Medicine published a case where a 59-year old woman with ARMD used nutrition along with chelation for her condition. After undergoing the recommended series of chelation, her vision improved to 20/25 in one eye and 20/20 in the other. Her central vision was greatly enhanced. One year later, her vision improvement remained.

Dr. Merrill Lipton of Belton, Texas, tells a compelling story of his experience with chelation and macular degeneration.

> I was injured during World War II, at the age of twenty, by an explosion above my head. Large pieces of shrapnel lodged in my head, near my ear and behind my eye. This left me with increased pressure in my right eye, which

resulted in glaucoma. Several years later, the same condition developed in my left eye. It was controlled with drops. In 1991, I thought I had cataracts. It turned out to be macular degeneration. I took forty chelation treatments and continued with follow-up treatments twice a month. My vision returned to 20/20 with correction, and my high blood pressure of twenty years' standing was cured. A few years later, I had my cataract removed, and complications resulted in increased intra occular pressure again. Back on chelation, this problem resolved to the extent that, at seventy-five years of age, I read without glasses and drive.

The word "chelation" is taken from the Greek work chele, meaning claw. This describes the way the molecules of the chelating agent grab onto the molecules of heavy metal, such as lead, iron, and copper, in the body and moves them to the kidneys, via the bloodstream, for excretion. The process of chelation also binds calcium, which is known, when it is present in cells in excessive amounts, to interfere with arterial health. Calcium is re sponsible for the build-up of plaque that causes blockages in the blood vessels. None of the calcium chelated and released during chelation is the calcium from bones and teeth. Chelation lowers serum ionized calcium which decreases clotting, reduces spasm and softens "hardening" of the arteries. A further benefit to overall health is that EDTA reduces the LDL cholesterol (the so-called 'bad' cholesterol) content in the liver and the plaque

How Chelation Works

Despite its success, scientists do not know for certain how chelation works. One theory is that it reduces free radicals. As I explained in previous sections of this book, free radicals are the harmful by-products of metabolic processes. A related theory is that since heavy metals cause an increased production of free radicals, reducing them in the body reduces the numbers of free radicals. Yet another understanding of how chelation works focuses on the relationship between calcium and magnesium as intracellular and intercellular components. As excess calcium is bound in the bloodstream, the calcium/ magnesium balance is favorably affected.

Finding a Doctor for Chelation

The ACAM maintains a list of doctors who are trained and certified to administer chelation therapy. The actual certification is done by the American Board of Chelation Therapy. This group monitors the preparation for this recognized medical subspecialty. It is important for you to work with such an individual. Unfortunately chelation therapy is not recognized by the medical profession as an accepted treatment. Beyond this, there are physicians who erroneously believe that it is harmful, or, at best, not useful. They will surely discourage their patients from using it. In the case of ARMD, however, they will also tell their patients that nothing can be done. You will most likely need to begin your own advocacy program for your vision as well as your overall health. Why wait and let precious time pass when there are effective techniques you can use to imrove your sight?

Medical science is notoriously slow to recognize and approve methods that have arisen outside the pharmaceutical/technology world. These giant profit-making businesses have quite a grip on the world of health care. They control research and virtually all innovation. Doctors have a hard time evaluating techniques that do not arise within this monolith. However, since most of them refuse to do their own research in chelation, they are not in a position to evaluate it. You can do this for yourself, however. A good starting point is requesting information from ACAM. The books by Dr. Morton Walker are also very valuable sources. He describes chelation from a scientific as well as case study perspective.

The next two chapters introduce two additional therapies for you to consider in your efforts to reverse your ARMD. Please read them before you choose which therapy to use. Of course, you can combine two or even all three if you wish. Chelation is the most expensive of the therapies, but it is invaluable if you have circulatory problems in addition to ARMD. Most important is choosing at least one of these approaches to healing your ARMD!

Checklist For Step Nine

√ Contact ACAM to learn more about chelation therapy.

√ Determine whether there is a doctor in your community who practices chelation.

√ Have a general checkup to evaluate your cardiovascular health.

Step 10

Homeopathy: Heal from Within

In this chapter, I will introduce you to one of the most dynamic and easy-to-use methods of total healing – homeopathy. By total healing, I mean that homeopathy can heal your mental attitude, emotional state, as well as your physical disease. I have seen it work absolute wonders for my patients regardless of their eye condition. For those with macular degeneration, it offers hope for great improvement in vision as well as in transforming one's attitude about the condition. Patients with ARMD who have taken a homeopathic remedy not only notice improved vision, but they report being calmer, more peaceful, less irritable, and able to enjoy the normal activities of life fully. They no longer focus on how their condition limits them but feel restored to a sense of gratitude for all that life offers. It is with a deep sense of commitment to this form of healing that I speak to you about homeopathy. I hope you will read this with an attitude of hope and interest and will consider homeopathy in your healing journey.

Homeopathy

What is Homeopathy?

Homeopathy is a natural system of healing based on the principle that 'like cures like.' This means that the symptoms of a disease resemble the symptoms that might be brought on in a healthy person who took a particular herb or other substance. One good example is with the remedy, mercury. When healthy people take an overdose of mercury and endured mercury poisoning, they experience tremors, excessive salivation, and an exquisite sensitivity to temperature change. When sick people, perhaps those with the flu, exhibit these symptoms, they will likely be cured if they take homeopathic mercury. In another example, we can look at how women in the past century took a little of the plant "belladonna"(it means pretty lady) in order to bring color to their cheeks and brightness to their eyes. Belladonna happens to be the homeopathic remedy one would think of using if a person had a fever accompanied by a bright red face and glistening eyes.

While this is the underlying principle of homeopathy, it does not tell us how it works. In fact, we don't know how it works. Homeopathic remedies, in addition to matching the person's symptoms, are made from minute doses of the substance used to heal those symptoms. The doses are so tiny that, at some strength, the substance cannot even be detected in a chemical analysis of the remedy. And these strengths, called the high potencies, are the most powerful in their ability to heal! Some feel that homeopathy is a type of energy medicine- one that works on the non-material levels of the person. Others feel that we cannot measure the substance because our instruments are not that subtle yet. Regardless of how it works, the important thing for me and for you is to know that it does work.

Homeopathic Remedies

Homeopathic remedies are made from plants, animals, and minerals. Belladonna is an example of a plant remedy, while mercury is an example of a mineral source. Most animal remedies are made from insects, snake venom, or the milk of mammals. There are about 3000 remedies. The key to success in homeopathy is selecting the correct remedy. While it is true that about three dozen remedies cover a wide variety of illnesses and will help a large number of people, it is still important to consider all the remedies when prescribing for a case. Remedies come in two forms. The dry form, or pellets, consists of small sugar pills taken by mouth under the tongue. This form is very easy and pleasant to take. Equally pleasant, but a little more complex is taking a liquid form of the remedy. These are prescribed by homeopaths, and, if you should need one, he or she will give you instructions. Unlike prescription or even over-the-counter drugs, remedies are taken for a short time only. In fact, you may only need one dose of a remedy to have a profound healing response. This is because of the way remedies work.

Remedies come in different strengths, called potencies. These cover a very wide range of strengths. The remedies available in health food stores are in the low to low-mid range in potency. Higher potencies, which are almost always needed to heal a serious chronic or degenerative condition, are available only by prescription through a homeopaths. Although I do not suggest that you try to self treat your ARMD, I do suggest that you go to a health food store and look at the section with homeopathic remedies. You will probably see several types of remedies. One type may be labeled according to a disease or conditions, such as "arthritis" or "sinus" or "indigestion." These may be either tablets or tinctures which are liquid forms. They will contain a number of remedies, and, thus, are called combination remedies. I consider these somewhat useful for people to get acquainted with homeopathy, but they do not in any way represent the full power of homeopathy.

Most likely you will also see some single remedies with unfamiliar names. These are likely to be packaged in small tubes. Inside are tiny white pellets. These are the most familiar and frequently used homeopathic remedies. People with some experience and knowledge of homeopathy use these to treat themselves, their families, and their pets. Although I strongly advise you to consult a skilled homeopathic practitioner to treat your ARMD, you may find these remedies useful for other conditions.

How do Remedies Work

Homeopathic remedies work to stimulate your own vital force, or immune response, to heal your illness. Although they are taken in a form that resembles regular medicine, they are completely different. For example if you had a bacterial infection such as a strep throat, the antibiotics you might take would actually kill the germs that caused the infection. However, if you were to take a homeopathic remedy for that same condition, the remedy would stimulate your own immune system to overcome the germs. And it would do this without causing any side effects whatsoever.

Another way remedies differ from regular medicine is in their timing. Many prescription drugs need to accumulate in your system before they can affect it. Antidepressants are one example. A person often needs to take an anti-depressant for several weeks before it has any effect. In homeopathy, there is no such thing as a cumulative effect. You can take one dose of a remedy and have an immediate effect. Or you can take one dose and have an effect several days or weeks later without taking any more doses. This is because the remedy works deeply in your system to mobilize your own healing forces. People who have been seriously ill and/or ill for a long time may require a longer period before they notice a response to a remedy. They may also require a repeated dose in a few months' time. A homeopath will carefully observe your response to the remedy and determine the potency and frequency of repetition.

Homeopathic Remedies may have an immediate effect.

Homeopathy

The Power of Homeopathy

One of the reasons why I have dedicated so much of my life and my practice to homeopathy is because of its power. It can cure disease states at every level of seriousness. For example, it is very effective in what we call 'acute' illness. This means short term intense diseases like flu, fever, pneumonia, and some injuries. It is also highly effective in curing chronic illness such as asthma, arthritis, lupus, and eye conditions. It can help where conventional medicine has nothing to offer besides powerful medications like steroids that do so much harm to the body while they relieve symptoms. It is also excellent at resolving deep emotional states such as anxiety, unexpressed or lingering grief, and depression. Mental/emotional disorders like panic attacks and attention deficit disorder respond beautifully. Even when people have terminal illness and organ changes that make it impossible for them to recover, homeopathy can relieve their pain as well as bring peace to their final days.

One dramatic story is the apparent reversal of a very severe and acute condition called central retinal arterial occlusion. Dr. Sobhendranath Datta, a radiologist from Louisiana, was attending a conference in my city when he was struck with what he called a "blackout in the left eye." His vision was better in the dark and very poor in light. He consulted me on an emergency basis, and I was able to prescribe a homeopathic remedy that restored his vision to 20/30. When he visited his doctor for a follow-up, the doctor said he had never seen an occlusion improve like that. 'He told me that, without homeopathic treatment, I would have lost sight in that eye. I got my vision back 100 percent with homeo-pathic medicine. This is a miracle. I am very grateful to you, Dr. Kondrot. I am blessed indeed.'

The Origin of Homeopathy

You may be wondering where this powerful healing system originated. You may also be wondering why it is not used more often and accepted as part of standard medicine. Samuel Hahnemann (1754-1840?) who was born in Germany is considered the father of homeopathy. While it is based on ancient healing systems as well as folk knowledge and herbal medicine, many aspects of it are entirely his original contribution. The idea of using a minute dose was never applied so effectively or systematically before Hahnemann. It is interesting to note that many modern doctors are using fractional or small doses of chemotherapy in place of the massive doses formerly given. And this is having very good results without the debilitating side effects.

Hahnemann was trained as a medical doctor, but was appalled at the harm done by the standard practices of the time. For example, many patients died from mercury poisoning and blood letting. On the other hand,

153

simple folk remedies, while they did no harm, were not powerful enough to cure serious diseases. He set about finding a new system and applied his considerable intellect and scientific training to do so. By the time of his death in the mid nineteenth century, homeopathy had spread throughout Europe, to North and South America, and to Asia. At the turn of the century about half of US medical schools trained homeopathic doctors. Homeopathy had its demise in the US as a result of the growth of the pharmaceutical companies. There is virtually no opportunity to make large profits in the manufacture of homeopathic remedies. Homeopathy also did not lend itself to standardized research for a number of reasons. So, with the growth in power of conventional medicine, homeopathy went 'underground' until its rebirth about twenty-five years ago. There are now many fine training programs operating in the US as well as abroad and the number of qualified homeopaths is increasing yearly.

Choosing a Homeopath

Many people purport to practice homeopathy, but , in my opinion, only some of these people are qualified to do so. I am going to give you guidelines to use in selecting a homeopath if you decide to do so. A homeopath may or may not be trained in another medical profession. Some homeopaths are MDs, some are chiropractors, naturopaths or acupuncturists. Some are simply trained as homeopaths. What you should look for is a classically trained homeopath who is certified by the

Council for Homeopathic Certification and uses the letters CCH after their name. These individuals have passed a test that indicates the high level of their competence. They have also met the Council's rigorous standard with respect to their education.

The National Center for Homeopathy maintains a list of practicing homeopaths throughout the US. This organization makes no claims about the competence of those it lists, but is a good place to start if you do not know how to find a homeopath in your area. The phone number is listed under references. Finally you can visit the website of the Hahnemann College of Homeopathy which maintains a list of its graduates. I can vouch for the quality of their training since that is where I received mine.

Their website is www/hahnemanncollege.org.

A Homeopathic Consultation

A visit to a homeopath is quite different than an appointment with a regular doctor. First of all, the homeopath will be interested in many things about you that an ordinary doctor would ignore. Homeopaths consider the way that you think, feel, look, as well as how your particular illness affects you as part of the symptoms that will help them find the correct remedy for you. To a homeopath, everything about a person expresses who they are and what medicine they might need. For example, your tendency to be warm or chilly as well as food preferences are important in understanding your case.

Homeopathy

Even if a homeopath saw three people with ARMD in one day, they would focus on the unique aspects of each person's situation. One person might be quite passive in accepting their diagnosis while another might be very anxious. One person might fear that their eye condition was a sign of other underlying disease, while another might feel grateful that they had only an eye condition. Similarly, one person might have insomnia or anxiety at night while another sleeps soundly but awakens with a headache almost every day. All of these distinctions would be important to the homeopath. Along with these characteristics, the homeopath might ask about your childhood and your dreams.

Many people report that their visit to a homeopath is one of the most enjoyable experiences that they have had. The visit usually takes from one to two hours and is conducted in an atmosphere free of judgment. The homeopath's focus is completely on the client and on anything he or she wants to discuss. There is no pressure to discuss things that make the client uncomfortable.

Shortly after the visit, the homeopath will prescribe a remedy and will tell the client how to obtain it. The next appointment will probably be in four to six weeks. At that time the homeopath will assess how well the remedy has worked. He or she may or may not prescribe another remedy at that time. In terms of expectations, it is important for patients to know that long term chronic conditions may take a while to resolve fully. A rule of thumb is that one month is required to heal a person for each year they have had the disease. All the while the remedy is working deeply and the person's underlying state is being strengthened.

One of my patients illustrates the mind/body effect of homeopathy very well. He is a young man who has had retinitis pigmentosis since he was a boy. He is both artistic and athletic but his diminished peripheral vision makes it difficult for him to enjoy these activities. He is a loner by nature but would like to have more satisfying relationships. When I first saw him, I was aware of a deep sadness about him, although he was quite unemotional in the consultation. As he opened up I discovered that he was quite depressed, and that he was preoccupied with thoughts of death.

I prescribed a remedy that is well known to help people release grief and other strong emotions when they are held in. Since taking his prescription, he has had many dreams with emotional content. He has also decided that he wants more satisfying social contacts and has developed a lot of insight into how he sabotages possibilities in these areas. He is less moody, more active, and more interested in pursuing other lifestyle changes that will improve his vision.

Homeopathy and ARMD

I have treated many patients who have ARMD with homeopathy. And I recommend that after proper nutrition and vitamin therapy patients immediately begin homeopathic treatment. Many patients will notice an immediate improvement of vision; others will notice a slow improvement over several months. Most patients will experience an improvement of their well being and out-

Homeopathy

look. Many other ailments, such as arthritis, will also improve under homeopathic treatment.

There is a long history of treating eye conditions with homeopathy. For about seventy years, from 1870 to 1940, the College of the New York Ophthalmic Hospital offered postgraduate courses in homeopathic ophthalmology. During this same period, there was a medical society devoted to homeopathy and ophthalmology and two journals published in the US. From 1870 to 1916, twelve major works on the homeopathic treatment of eye diseases were published. Many cases were published in the literature of the time, showing improvement in a variety of eye diseases. These were all the more remarkable since there were no other treatments available at the time for serious eye disorders. Because this is still true with macular degeneration, homeopathy is a vitally important part of therapy for this condition.

I urge you to consider homeopathic treatment along with implementing the lifestyle changes described in the earlier chapters of this book. Homeopathy is also compatible with chelation therapy and micro current stimulation. You can do all of these to give yourself a comprehensive healing experience as well as maximize your chance to reverse your ARMD.

Checklist for Step Ten

√ Visit a health food store and look at the
homeopathic remedy section.

√ Purchase something for your own use,
such as Arnica spray for injuries or
Calendula ointment for cuts.

√ Contact the National Center for Homeopathy and determine whether there
is a homeopath in your area.

Homeopathy

Step 11

Microcurrent
Stimulation:
Wake up your Eyes

After treatment with Microcurrent Stimulation I left the office that same day with
my vision improved to 20/25. I could legally drive again. As important as that
is, with the use of Microcurrent Stimulation at home, my vision has remained
the same for more than nine months
now. Please let everyone who can benefit from this treatment know that there
is hope.   B.J.C., Naples, Florida

In this chapter, I am going to introduce you to one
of the most revolutionary treatments for ARMD. It is
called Microcurrent Stimulation, and it consists of applying weak current to the energy, or acupressure, points
that encircle the eye on the bony ridge.

I have been using Microcurrent Stimulation since Au-
gust of 1998 and have been very impressed with the improvement I have seen in the vision of patients with
ARMD. Most patients will begin to see an improvement
after 4 days of treatment. This is a therapy that can be
done at home with some simple instructions. The physi-

Microcurrent Stimulation

cians using this device, myself included, are seeing a measurable improvement in 70% of their patients. Microcurrent stimulation uses equipment similar to that used by doctors and in hospitals on a daily basis to help with pain management, bone regeneration, and healing transplanted tissue. You may have known someone with a bad backache who was given a TENS (Transcutaneous Electrical Nerve Stimulation) Unit to wear for a while. Or perhaps you have heard of someone who suffered a severe fracture and was given a TENS unit to stimulate healing of the plates of the bones. Grace Halloran (author of *Amazing Grace* and vision therapy instructor) used it to help heal her 8-year-old son's elbow fracture after doctors told her the arm would not grow because the plates were damaged. "He recovered completely, and is now a grown man...with two equal arms." Encouraged by this, she began to use it on her eyes. "Soon I realized my sight was getting better, both at night and in my field of vision."

In the same way that chelation therapy uses a chemical substance for another purpose than its main medical application, Microcurrent Stimulation uses a device similar to the TENS for another purpose. Microcurrent Stimulation devices are available through my office and from the manufacturer and inventor, Joel Rossen. His phone number and website are listed in the Resoures section. The devices are patented and approved for marketing by the FDA. However, you need a physician's prescription to get one. This is not because they are dangerous but because we feel that patients need to be trained and supported in their use.

Using the Microcurrent Stimulation 100 device is not only painless, it is experienced as pleasant by most patients. The technique involves touching an electrode, which is the size and shape of a pencil, to points on the bony ridge around your eye. The patient is always in control of the level of current, and the best results are obtained when virtually no current is perceptible. The device is very easy to use. Replacement and upgraded parts are readily available from the manufacturer.

> The macular specialists can give only negative advice, but not one...had a treatment to improve my vision with Microcurrent Stimulation the improvement so far has been that I can read an additional line on the chart, but further, my general vision is clearer and brighter. I am greatly encouraged.
> R.L.R., Boynton Beach, Florida

The theory behind the effectiveness of microcurrent stimulation is that our cells are like batteries. When we age or develop a degenerative disease, these batteries become incapable of retaining their proper charge. They need to be stimulated just as a car battery does when it is 'dead' with the current from another source. The flow of current from cell to cell and within cells promotes repair and regeneration of tissue. In ARMD, it promotes the flushing away of toxins while energizing the tissues of the retina and macula. You will recall that dry ARMD is characterized by the accumulation of residue in the macula when circulation is inadequate to remove it.

Microcurrent Stimulation

The devices used for ocular stimulation in conditions such as ARMD, retinitis pigmentosa, cataract, and glaucoma was designed and patented by Joel Rossen. He is the inventor of the Microcurrent Stimulation Unit used for eye disease. The unit comes in a package about the size of a small handbag. All components are neatly packaged, and the instructions are very clear. Patients who are able to visit an ophthalmologist's office for their initial instruction and start-up treatments should do so. They will then follow this series with home treatments twice daily. The treatments take about 15 minutes to complete.

How Does Microcurrent Stimulation Work?

There are several metabolic processes that are enhanced through the use of Microcurrent Stimulation. The first is to boost the cells' ability to rid themselves of waste products. A cell with 'stuck' waste products becomes a dead cell and interferes with cellular communication throughout the area where it is located. Cells need to take in nutrients and eliminate waste like every other living organism. The energy supplied by Microcurrent Stimulation allows cells to become more vital and less sluggish in doing so. The second way Microcurrent Stimulation works is by increasing the blood supply to the area stimulated. A simple study measuring the size of blood vessels before and after treatment showed that virtually all blood vessels were larger after treatment. This demonstrates how this therapy brings a new blood supply to the area to nourish and refresh cells and tissues.

Microcurrent Stimulation was also shown to relax muscles in the treated area. This, of course, also paves the way for increased nutrition and oxygenation of tissues. In macular degeneration, the retinal cells are sick and not functioning properly. The electrical current gently wakes up the cells from sleep and stimulates the healing process.

The Body Electric

It may come as a surprise to you to know that prior to the early part of this century, healing through the use of electric therapy was quite well-accepted. As the world of medicine became more focused on proof and scientific explanations, biochemistry came to dominate the form of treatment. We must not overlook the fact that this coincided with the dawn of an era where synthetic chemical products, including drugs, were first developed. Interestingly, chemical formulas are based on an understanding of atomic theory – that matter is composed of atoms that have components that are both positive and negatively charged. Chemical bonding is the result of atoms attempting to stabilize themselves by combining with other atoms. It makes sense, then, to postulate that all of life is composed of 'charged' matter. This includes the human body, all of its tissues, cells, and fluids.

When atoms combine with each other, they exchange electrons, the negatively charged outer elements in their shell. This flow of electrons from one atom to another is called current and it goes on continuously in our bodies as well as other living forms. Some scientists believe that there are specialized cells that are responsible for conducting current. These cells form rapidly at the site of an injury in order to promote healing. Studies have measured an increase in positive charge at injury and amputation sites. This tends to return to negative after healing is underway. The theory is that the charge attracts healing forces in the body to congregate at the injury site. When researchers have attempted to manipulate the flow of electricity to injury sites, they have repeatedly discovered that a low current is the most useful to enhance healing. In fact, a strong current can disrupt it. That is why, in Microcurrent Stimulation, the flow of current is imperceptible.

Treatment Protocol

Patients who want to use microcurrent stimulation first need a complete eye examination. The dry type of ARMD responds better to microcurrent stimulation although many patients with the wet form also notice a significant improvement. Patients with vision better than 20/400 vision (being able to barely see the big "E" on the eye chart) also respond better to treatment although I have seen dramatic improvement in patients with worse vision.

> Sam Snead, 85-year old professional golfer, announced his return to golf and intention to obtain a driver's license after undergoing Microcurrent Stimulation treatment for his macular degeneration. His vision went from 20/100 to 20/30 in

one eye after a course of treatment.

Patients receive eight office treatments with the microcurrent stimulation unit over a one week period. Then they receive instructions on the home unit and begin treatment twice a day for 3 months. After that the treatments are reduced to once a day for 3 months and then several times a week to maintain the level of vision. Special glasses are being developed that will make self-treatment even easier. They will be an all-in-one unit that targets the acupuncture points near the eyes and provides the stimulation simply by putting them on.

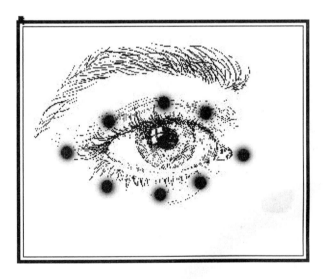

THIS SHOWS THE MAJOR ACUPRESSURE POINTS LOCATED AROUND THE EYE

It is also important to begin vitamin and mineral

therapy during Microcurrent Stimulation treatment. All patients in my practice begin the macular degeneration formula (two tablets three times a day) and the **Pure Focus**™ spray three times a day.

Research

One study that included patients with ARMD showed impressive results. The average improvement for patients who used Microcurrent Stimulation for two to seven years was 2.125 additional letters read on the Snellen chart. Patients also reported that their vision was brighter. A similar group who did not receive microcurrent stimulation treatment had a loss of 7.1 letters over the same time period.

No discussion of Microcurrent Stimulation would be complete without mention of the pioneering work of John Jarding, an optometrist in Hot Springs, South Dakota. His search for a way to help his patients with ARMD led him to begin this work over ten years ago, when very few had heard of it. He presented it to the scientific community and many of us have been very active in attempting to bring this technique into mainstream medical care.

Is Microcurrent Stimulation for You?

It is hard not be impressed with the results of this treatment, especially for a condition regarded as hopeless by conventional medicine. You may well be wondering if this is something for you to consider doing. I would like to offer this guidance. People who have had serious deterioration, so that their vision is 20/400 or worse, may not have good results with this treatment. Those with wet form ARMD who have had bad effects from laser surgery will not be able to be helped. However, if they have one eye that has not had this trauma, they may get results in that eye. Those who are newly diagnosed and have a small loss in acuity will most likely respond the best. Individuals who have had cataract surgery should consider this therapy since ARMD often follows cataract surgery. The next thing to consider is your commitment. Once you embark on Microcurrent Stimulation therapy and have realized improvement in your vision, you will need to continue doing it several times weekly. Those who have stopped the therapy have had their vision deteriorate. However, once you own the unit and learn the technique, this is not a hardship

The price of the unit is around $700, although this can vary depending on how you obtain it. This is a one time purchase and it includes all the equipment needed for years of use. As of this writing, neither Medicare nor private insurance pays for the device or the treatment.

The wife of one of my patients (JS) writes this after her husband visited my office for his initial set of Microcurrent Stimulation treatments. Fortunately, I hear good news like this quite often.

We left for Florida the next day. Along the way he began to see the trees alongside the car on the highway. Later he saw a car ahead of us about 150 feet away. Since that day he has been able to see things on a day-at-a-time basis. He saw his face in a mirror, made a phone call with no help, and can pick out numbers on a calculator. He still sits close to the TV, but he can see many more details. He saw the red and green on a stoplight. Jack's distance vision, thus far, has progressed faster than his close vision. But, as he says, 'If it never progresses any farther... but holds where it is right now, he'll be the happiest man on earth.' We, and all our friends, are amazed and so excited. Everyone wants to know who our doctor is.... So, if your phone rings off the wall, it's probably someone we've given your number to. Thank you for trying when the other specialists told us, 'Nothing can be done for ARMD at this time.'

A.S., New Port Richey Florida.

I have now explained three treatments for ARMD. These are homeopathy, chelation therapy, and Microcurrent Stimulation. At this step in the process of your healing, you need to select one of these as the final phase of your program to reverse your ARMD. You may find, eventually, that you can benefit from two or maybe all three techniques. Variables for this include the severity of your condition, the proximity of doctors who offer these treatments, and the amount of time and money you can spend. I urge you not to deprive yourself of these simple and effective techniques. The next chapter offers a review of the material in this book as a way to solidify your program.

Microcurrent Stimulation

Step 12

Put it All Together: 90 Days to Better Vision

Hopefully this book has challenged you to assume control of your vision – and your overall health. Having done this, you will want to set goals for yourself – and begin to make choices—some small, some large—that will move you toward your goals. I urge you to make haste slowly. Make haste because your condition is one that, left alone, will deteriorate steadily. The sooner you begin a program to reverse it, the better. Go slowly in the sense of not feeling overwhelmed. Remember, managing stress applies to this process also.

You may have noticed that this book is divided into three main sections. The first four chapters urge you to take charge of your health through assertiveness, improved diet, an exercise program, and stress reduction. The second section targets your eyes by recommending exercises and relaxation for them as well as specific foods, supplements, and herbal additions to your diet. You might say that this is a second level or higher degree of commitment. Then, in the last three chapters, I explained, in detail, three therapies that zone in on your ARMD in a treatment sense. All of this may seem a little overwhelm-

173

ing. That is why I recommend a ninety day time period to 'phase in' all the aspects of your personal plan for healing your vision. And, yes, I suggest you take thirty days for each of the sections.

The First Month

The work you do in developing a program based on the recommendations of the first four chapters will pay off handsomely in more ways than you can imagine just yet. A sound healthful diet, regular exercise, and learning a way to relax are keys to a vital, satisfying life. But we are actually going to start at the beginning

In the first chapter, I challenged you to inform yourself about your condition. You would be amazed at the number of patients I see who have no idea what their diagnosis is or when their condition began. I want you to position yourself squarely in charge of your health and your vision. Sure, you can and should use doctors and specialists of all sorts to help you recover. But use them like consultants. Listen to their advice and compare it to all the other information you have, including the information in this book. Do not hand over your power to your doctor. If you were buying a new kitchen appliance or a new car, would you just tell the salesperson to give you whatever they thought you needed? Of course not. Yet, when it comes to our health and our bodies we are very apt to be cowed into submission by the authority of a doctor. Therefore, I suggest that you listen carefully to your *diagnosis* and forget whatever your doctor says about your *prognosis*. Once you take your healing into your own hands, you are the only authority about it.

Reshape Your Eating Habits

I have laid it our pretty clearly in the second chapter. Now you need the motivation to do it. You have a serious degenerative disease. This means that, at some level, your body has a toxic overload. Start to clean up your act. While I emphasized what to add, (you will be quite busy eating daily servings of greens among your five servings of organic produce) you may need to concentrate on giving some things up. Eliminate the following foods from your diet as rapidly as possible. They are at best empty calories and at worst absolutely harmful to the health of your eyes—and the rest of you.

Coffee Margarine Hydrogenated fat products Desserts Processed foods Fast foods Soft drinks	Give These Up!

Select your form of exercise and get going. Reread the section on rebounding on a trampoline. This is so easy, convenient, economical, and fun. Its health benefits are enormous. You may be a person who likes a gym environment. Join one and figure out how and when you are going to get there. Walking is easy. Race walking is even more beneficial for the time involved. Make exercise a new and positive addiction to take the place of some of the negative ones listed above.

Begin to relax on a daily basis. Yoga combines exercise and relaxation. In the beginning, you may need to think about efficiencies like this so that you touch base on all these points in the first 30 days. Whenever you balk at all these changes, consider the alternative. Consider helplessly watching your sight deteriorate over the next few years until you cannot see the faces of loved ones, go anywhere alone, and become a burden to your family. The prospect of such a limited life should be motivation!

The Second Month

With the basics of diet, exercise, and relaxation in place, you are now ready to design your focused eye health program. The focus is on your eyes of course, and the program has four parts.

Part One means beginning a daily routine of eye relaxation and exercise. As your overall health and circulation improves through the changes you made in the first month, it is time to take some of the nourishment directly to your eyes. Palming can become a part of your relaxation program with virtually no effort at all. The other techniques are easy to do and do not require much time. The challenge is to remember to do them. But, you are becoming an expert at change already.

Part two requires you to add the lutein and zeaxanthin containing foods we talked about in the sixth chapter. With a great new diet under your belt, adding these daily is like frosting on the cake. Remember cake? Find your favorites among the greens and work them into each day's food intake. Even if you eat nothing else, eat your greens.

Clear some counter space for your **Pure Focus™** and the vitamin/mineral supplements I've outlined for you. Look around for the most effective and efficient way to take them. The fewer pills and capsules the better.

Be certain that the wonderful eye herbs – bilberry, gingko, and eyebright are among your supplements. In some cases you can find these as ingredients in high quality eye formulas. If not, then you will need to buy and take them separately.

The Third Month

Now it is time to choose a first technique to try and heal your vision. You are stronger and healthier now from the good diet and exercise. You are more relaxed too. Perhaps a direction has come to you during one of your relaxation sessions. The body knows what is good for it. As you detoxify and build up through better nutrition, you will find yourself able to make better choices in all areas of your life. It is time to choose to begin chelation therapy, homeopathy, or microcurrent stimulation. You do not need to limit yourself to one of these, but you will probably want to begin with one.

Chelation is a good choice if you have heart or circulatory problems in addition to your ARMD. This is another one of those overall health enhancing choices. Unfortunately you may not be able to find a doctor in your
area who does chelation. Chelation does require a considerable outlay of time and money since many sessions are
required. However, if it helps you avoid an invasive surgical procedure for your heart disease it is priceless.

Homeopathy is an excellent choice if you feel that
negative mental/emotional states are part of your overall approach to life. It will also be able to help with chronic
conditions, tendencies and weaknesses you have had since
birth, hormonal problems, and energy and sleep difficulties. Of course, homeopathy can be combined with
chelation and microcurrent stimulation. If there is no
homeopath in your area, you might be able to find one
who will work on a telephone consultation basis, after
one visit, or in place of a visit. The important thing is to
pursue this if it resonates with you.

Microcurrent stimulation is something I recommend
for all patients with ARMD. After the initial payment for
the equipment, there are no additional fees. It is something that you can do at home, on your own schedule,
and forever if you choose. You can order your unit while
you are looking for a source for chelation and/or homeopathy.

I have just told you how to revolutionize your life
and overcome a lifetime of bad habits in three months. I
hope you believe in yourself enough to do this. I hope
you have whatever support you need to assume responsibility for reversing your ARMD. I have tried to give you

the tools and the encouragement that you will not find anywhere else. Please take these gifts and use them to heal yourself in mind, body, and spirit.

TWELVE STEPS TO BETTER VISION

1. Eat Well

2. Exercise your Body

3. Control Stress

4. Supplement Your Diet

5. Eat for your sight

6. Use Herbs for your eyes

7. Exercise Your Eyes

8. Choose a therapy:

    9. Chelation

    10. Homeopathy

    11. Microcurrent Stimulation

12. *Put it All Together!*

RESOURCES - **Chapter One**

The Amsler Grid

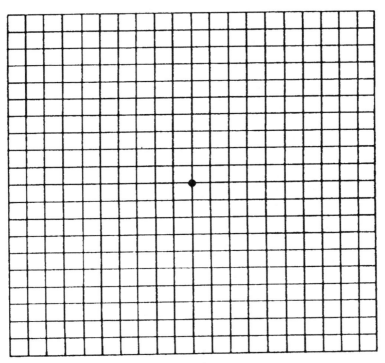

Instructions
1. Sit in good light; put on your reading or near glasses
2. Hold the grid 12 inches from your eyes
3. Cover the left eye and look directly at the black dot
4. While looking at the dot, look at the grid pattern with your side vision. Note any missing or distorted lines or gray areas.
   Mark these with a pencil.
5. Cover the right eye and repeat # 3 and 4.

RESOURCES
Chapter Four
Books

Bates, W. H., M.D., *The Cure of Imperfect Sight by Treatment Without Glasses* (New York:Central Fixation Publishing, 1920)

Pelletier, Kenneth, *Mind As Healer, Mind As Slayer,* Delacorte Press, 1977

Selye, Hans, *Stress Without Distress,* New American Library, 1974

Chapter Five
Books

Mansfield, Peter, *The Bates Method,* Vermilion Press, London, 1992

Schneider, Meir, *My Life and Vision,* Viking Penguin, New York, 1987

Organizations

The American Vision Institute
referral to vision training specialists
1111 Howe Street
Sacramento CA 95825
(916) 929-8831

The Bates Teachers Association
referral and teacher training
Vision Training Institute
11303 Meadow View Road
El Cajon CA 920

RESOURCES
Chapter Six
> To order **Pure Focus**™
> **Nutritional Research LLC**
> www.nutritionalresearch.net
> (toll free) 1-877-341-2703

Chapter Seven
> Books
> Haas, Elson, *Staying Healthy with Nutrition*, Berkeley,
>   Celestial Arts, 1992
> Murray, Michael ND & Pizzorno, Joseph ND,
>   *Encyclopedia of Natural Medicine*, Rocklin, CA,
>   Prima Publishing, 1991

> To order Macular Degeneration Formula
> Nutritional Research LLC
> www.nutritionalresearch.net
> (toll free) 1-877-341-2703

Chapter Nine
> ACAM
> American College of Advancement in Medicine
> 1-800/ 532-3688
> referral to doctors who use chelation therapy

RESOURCES
Chapter Ten
Referral
National Center for Homeopathy
referral to homeopaths throughout the nation
(703) 548-7790
www.homeopathic.org)

Homeopathic Educational Resources
request their catalog of books on homeopathy.
1-800-359-9051

Hahnemann College of Homeopathy: for a list of
their graduates
www. hahnemanncollege.org

Books
Nauman, Eileen & Derin-Kellog, G. *Help and Home
opathy*, Cottonwood, AZ, Blue Turtle Publishing
Co, 1998
This is an excellent resource for using home
opathy in medical emergencies.

Schools
Hahnemann College
Point Richmond CA
(510) 232-2079
www.hahnemanncollege.org
A four-year program for licensed health
professsion.

RESOURCES

Desert Institute of Classical Homeopathy
Phoenix, AZ
(602) 347-7950
Contact Todd Rowe MD
2 program with clinical training

San Diego Center for Homeopathic
Education and Training
Escondido CA
(619) 260-1256

Chapter Eleven
Doctors who provide microcurrent stimulation training
and devices

Edward Kondrot MD
(412) 281-0447
1- 800 430-9328
239 4th ave Suite 2020
Pittsburgh PA 15222
www.homeopathiceye.com
ekondrot@pipeline.com
and
5501 N. 19th Ave Suite 425
Phoenix AZ 85015
(602) 347-7950

Damon Miller MD
881 Fremont Ave. Suite A5
Los Altos CA 94022
(650) 948-5120

RESOURCES

George Khouri MD
1411 N. Flagler Drive Suite 4100
West Palm Beach FL 33401
(561) 366-8300
www.palmbeacheye.com
email: info@palmbeach.com

Percival Chee MD
Kukui Plaza Mall Suite C 116
50 South Beretania Street
Honolulu HI 96813
(808) 521-6578

To find a doctor who uses Microcurrent Stimulation or to obtain a unit for your own use, contact:
Joel Rossen
1-800-326-9119
www. MicrocurrentStimulation.com

Healing the Eye

INDEX

G

Gamma linolenic acid, 120
Ginkgo biloba, 131
Glaucoma, 3
>Herbs, and, 128
>Microcurrent Stimulation, and 164

H

Hahnemann College of Homeopathy, 2, 184, 188
Hahnemann Medical School, 1, 188
Hahnemann, Samuel, 2
Halloran, Grace, 39, 102, 132, 162
Health Food Stores, 28-30
Herbs
>Active ingredient in, 128, 129
>Organic, 129
>Taking, 130
>Wildcrafted, 129
Hirsch, Dahlia, MD, xv, 22, 23, 34
Homeopathic remedies, 149-151
Homeopathy, 2, 147-158
>Eye condtions, and, 157, 158
>History of, 153
>Source for referral, 154, 184-185
Huxley, Aldous, 80
Hypertension, 10, 12, 23

I

Immune System, xii

About the Author

Edward Kondrot, MD received his medical degree from the Hahnemann Medical College in Philadelphia in 1977. He completed his training in ophthalmology at St. Francis Hospital in Pittsburgh and the Scheie Eye Institute in Philadelphia in 1981. He maintains practices in Pittsburgh, Pennsylvania and Phoenix, Arizona.

Dr. Kondrot has practiced homeopathy since 1990 and received a diploma from the Hahnemann College of Homeopathy in Point Richmond California in 1996. He contributed to the *Clinicians' Rapid Access Guide to Complementary and Alternative Medicine*, Mosby 2000, and has written numerous articles and conducted seminars for professional and lay audiences on the use of homeopathy, nutrition, microcurrent stimulation, and chelation therapy for diseases of the eye. He is recognized as a pioneer in the use of homeopathy for eye conditions and is on the faculty of the Desert Institute of Homeopathy in Phoenix, Arizona as well as at the San Diego Center for Homeopathic Education and Healing.

Dr. Kondrot can be reached at
1-800-430-9328
ekondrot@pipeline.com

www.homeopathiceye.com.

Notes

Notes

_____

Notes

Notes

_____

Notes

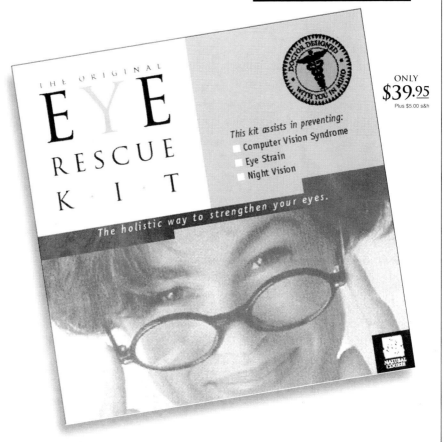

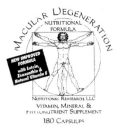
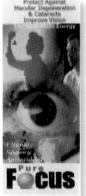